MW01283903

Your Family Pet-Treat Cookbook

Make all the dogs, cats and horses in your life happy by making special, wholesome treats for them right at home.

*Save money, while supporting
a great cause!*

Whitehall Publishing.
PO Box 548
Yellville, AR 72687
www.whitehallpublishing. com
E-mail info@whitehallpublishing.com

Whitehall Publishing is not responsible if the created recipe is fed in an irresponsible manner or if the animal reacts badly to a correctly prepared recipe. When introducing any new item into your animal's diet, start slowly and over the course of several days, increase the number of treats you are feeding your animal. Remember that these are "goodies"/special treats, not part of your animal's normal diet so feed them sparingly as you would with all treats. As always, when in doubt, consult your veterinarian.

$12.95
Printed in the USA

Table of Contents

TiP:

To avoid chubby pets, you should feed the fabulous treats in this book in small quantities until your pets get used to eating all-natural goodies.

Dogs, cats and horses can have finicky digestive systems and any change in their diet can result in an upset tummy, so start with no more than two treats per day and slowly work up to three a day, over the course of a week...
As always, when in doubt, consult your veterinarian!

About Us

Whitehall publishing is proud to support any individual or organization that is dedicated to helping those in need.

When you purchase this book, not only are you helping worthy causes within your community, but you are also going to save money when you create your own treats at home!

Don't forget that when you create your pet treats at home, you are using all natural ingredients with no preservatives and nothing is better for your pet then healthy food!

We encourage you to donate your time and talent to worthy organizations within your community who focus on helping those in need.

As is often the case in volunteering, your life will be richer for the experience!

Dog Treat Recipes

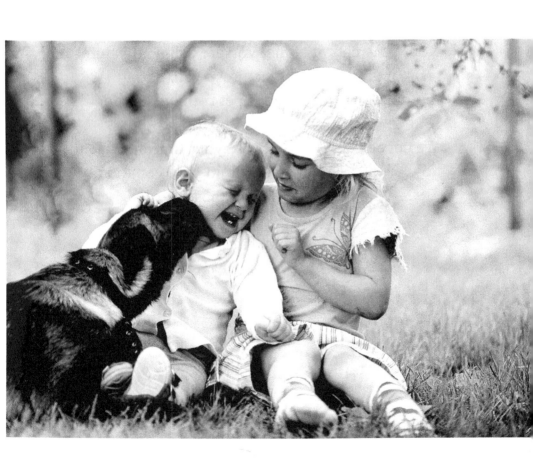

Beagle Bagels

1 cup whole wheat flour
1 cup unbleached flour
1 package yeast — 1/4 ounce
1 cup chicken broth — warmed
1 tablespoon honey
Preheat oven to 375 degrees.

1. In large bowl combine the whole wheat flour with the yeast.
2. Add 2/3 cup chicken broth and honey and beat for about 3 minutes.
3. Gradually add the remaining flour. Knead the dough for a few minutes until smooth and moist, but not wet (use reserve broth as necessary).
4. Cover the dough and let it rest for about 5 minutes.
5. Divide the dough into 15-20 pieces, rolling each piece into a smooth ball.
6. Punch a hole in each ball with your finger or end of spoon and gently pull the dough so the hole is about a 1/2" wide. Don't be too fussy here, the little bagels rise into shape when they bake.
7. Place on a greased cookie sheet and allow to rise for five minutes.
8. Bake for 25 minutes at 375 degrees.
9. Turn the heat off and allow the bagels to cool in the oven.

Paw Lickin' Liver Treats

1 pound beef liver
2 cloves garlic
1 box corn muffin mix
Preheat oven to temperature in corn muffin directions.

1. Mix liver and garlic in a blender or food processor, then process until liquid.
2. Stir in muffin mix, then scrape onto a baking sheet and pat to approximately 1/2 - 1" thickness.
3. Bake until very firm, but not burned, following the time directions on the corn muffin mix box.
4. Cut into squares, then store in refrigerator or freezer.

Heavenly Dog Biscuits

2	cups whole wheat flour	1/2	cup powdered milk
1	teaspoon salt	1/4	teaspoon garlic powder
1	egg	6	tablespoons vegetable oil
8	tablespoons water — (8 to 10)	2	jars babyfood, neat, beef, strained — *see Note

1. Mix all ingredients together and knead for 3 min. Roll out to 1 inch thick.Use a dog bone shaped cookie cutter, and place biscuits on an ungreased baking sheet.
2. Bake in preheated oven at 350 degrees for 20 to 25 min. Makes approximately 2 dozen doggie biscuits.

***Note:** Strain. Use beef, chicken or lamb.

Lovable Lhasa Apso Liver Brownies

1 pound chicken or beef liver
1/2 pound plain cornmeal (non-rising)
1/2 pound plain old-fashioned oatmeal
1 can salmon or mackerel (with juice)
1 cup chicken broth or water
1 tablespoon minced garlic
1 egg
1 dash of salt
1/4 cup parsley flakes

1. Place liver, egg, fish, broth, garlic, salt and parsley flakes in a blender or food processor and blend until smooth.
2. Mix corn and oat meal, and then add liver mixture.
3. Mix well.
4. Once mixed, batter should be like a slightly wet brownie mix.
5. Add more broth or water if necessary.
6. Pour mixture onto well-greased cookie sheet and bake at 250 degrees for 1 1/2 to 2 hours.
7. Cut into squares while still warm.
8. Cool, and then freeze what you won't use in one week or less.

Liver Treat Goodies

1 pound beef liver

All you need are beef livers. Try your local meat packers; they often throw them away. Or you can buy fresh liver from the supermarket.

1. Cut the liver into approximately 1 inch slices.
2. Place in your food dehydrator for 24 hours*. (Use Pam or the equivalent on the drying racks, so the liver won't stick. Let dry for 24 hours.)
*Or you could place them on a cookie sheet and bake in a 325 degree oven for about 45 minutes to help dry them out.

Yogurt Pups ala' Toto

16 ounces plain nonfat yogurt
3/4 cup water
1 tablespoon chicken bouillon granules

1. Dissolve bouillon in water.
2. Combine water and yogurt in blender and blend thoroughly.
3. Pour into small containers for freezing, cover and freeze.

Bacon Bites

3 cups whole wheat flour
1/2 cup milk
1 egg
1/4 cup bacon grease — or vegetable oil
1 teaspoon garlic powder
4 slices bacon — crumbled
1/2 cup cold water

1. Mix ingredients together thoroughly.
2. Roll out on a floured surface to 1/2 - 1/4" thickness. Cut into shapes and bake for 35-40 minutes in a 325 degree oven.

Blow Me Away Biscuits

3 1/2	cups flour	4	teaspoons salt
2	cups whole wheat flour	1/2	cup dry milk
1	cup rye flour	1	egg
1	cup cornmeal	1	package dry yeast (1 teaspoon)
2	cups cracked wheat	1	pint chicken stock

(Ingredients not generally available at grocery stores may be found at health food stores.)

1. Dissolve yeast in 1/4 cup warm water. Add chicken stock and pour into dry ingredients.
2. Knead for 3 minutes, working into a stiff dough. Roll dough into a 1/4" thick sheet and cut with cookie cutters (cutters shaped like dog biscuits are available).
3. Bake in 300 degree oven for 45 minutes, then turn oven off and leave biscuits in oven overnight. In the morning the biscuits will be bone hard.

Note: This dough is extremely stiff to work with, but the end product is excellent!

Rice Flour Canine Cookies

1 1/2 cups white rice flour
1 1/4 cups grated cheddar cheese
1/4 pound safflower oil — margarine
1 clove garlic — crushed

1. Grate the cheese and let stand until it reaches room temperature.
2. Cream the cheese with the softened margarine, garlic, and flour.
3. Add enough milk to form into a ball.
4. Chill for 1/2 hour.
5. Roll onto floured board.
6. Cut into shapes and bake at 375 degrees for 15 minutes or until slightly brown, and firm. Makes 2 to 3 dozen, depending on size.

Classic Canine Cookies

4 cups whole wheat flour
1/4 cup cornmeal
1/4 cup cooked rice
1 egg
2 tablespoons vegetable oil
Juice from a small orange
1 2/3 cups water

1. Mix all ingredients together well.
2. Turn out onto a lightly floured surface and knead. Roll out dough to about 1/8 inch thickness and cut out desired shapes (doggy bones, paws, balls, etc.)

Dipping Sauce:

#1
3 cups vanilla chips
1 tablespoon spinach powder
1 teaspoon garlic powder
1 teaspoon vegetable oil

#2
3 cups carob chips
1 teaspoon vegetable oil
1 teaspoon turmeric powder

1. Melt chips in a double boiler or microwave.
2. Add oils and seasonings.
3. Dip tips of cookies, when cooled, into desired sauce and place on a pan lined with wax paper until set.

Puppy Formulas

Recipe #1

2/3 cup goat's milk canned (or just regular canned milk)
1/3 cup water or Pedialyte
1 teaspoon Karo Syrup
1 egg yolk
1 teaspoon Dyne or pediatric vitamin

1. Strain a couple of times to make sure there is no albumin in the mixture, although it has been used successfully without egg at all.
Variation: 1 can of condensed milk rather than goat's milk (it may be too high in protein and put a strain on the puppy's kidneys 1 envelope of Knox unflavored gelatin in addition to other ingredients (helps keep stools solid).

Recipe #2

1 cup canned condensed milk or evaporated milk
4 ounces plain, full-fat yogurt
1 egg yolk
1 dropper full baby vitamins

1. Combine all ingredients and mix well before serving.

Recipe #3

2 cups hot water
1 can evaporated milk (Not condensed)
2 eggs
2 tablespoons Karo syrup
2 envelopes Knox unflavored gelatin.

1. Mix thoroughly to get the gelatin working.

Recipe #4

4 ounces Carnation evaporated milk
4 ounces full fat natural, plain yogurt
1 tablespoon mayonnaise,
1 egg yolk
1 dropper full human baby pediatric liquid vitamin

1. Mix in blender before serving.

Bulldog Brownies

Brownies:

1/2	cup shortening	3	tablespoons honey
4	eggs	1	teaspoon vanilla
1	cup whole wheat flour	1/4	cup carob flour
1/2	teaspoon baking powder		

Frosting:
12 ounces nonfat cream cheese
2 teaspoons honey

Brownies:
1. Cream shortening and honey together thoroughly.
2. Add remaining brownie ingredients. Beat well.
3. Bake in a greased cookie sheet (10x15") for 25 minutes at 350 degrees. Cool completely.

Frosting:
1. Blend frosting ingredients together.
2. Spread frosting over cool brownies.
3. Cut into 3 inch or 1 1/2 inch squares.

Boo Biscuits for Dogs

3 1/2	cup whole wheat flour	2	cup Quaker oats
1	cup milk	1/2	cup hot water
2	beef or chicken bouillon cubes	1/2	cup meat drippings

1. Dissolve bouillon cubes in hot water. Add milk and drippings and beat well.
2. In a separate bowl, mix flour and oatmeal.
3. Pour liquid ingredients into dry ingredients and mix well.
4. Press onto an ungreased cookie sheet and cut into shapes desired. Bake at 300 degrees for 1 hour.
5. Turn off heat and leave in the oven to harden. Refrigerate after baking.

Chicken Garlic Doggie Birthday Cake

1 chicken bouillon cube

2 cups wheat germ

2 eggs

1 tablespoon minced garlic
  vegetable oil spray — garlic flavor

1 cup whole-wheat flour

1/2 cup cornmeal

1/2 cup vegetable oil

2 cups water

Preheat oven to 375 degrees.

1. Dissolve bouillon cube in warm water.
2. Combine flour, wheat germ, cornmeal, eggs, oil, garlic and water.
3. Spray two cake pans with garlic-flavored oil, and sprinkle with flour.
4. Bake 50 minutes. After removing cake from oven, turn upside down and let cool. Makes two small cakes.

Special Lhasa Apso Lamb

1 pound lamb, ground — cooked

2 cups cooked white rice

4 cloves garlic — crushed

1/4 cup carrots, frozen — chopped

2 cups cooked brown rice

1 cup yogurt, (skim milk)

1/4 cup green beans, frozen — chopped

1/4 cup kale, frozen — chopped

1. Cook lamb and drain off excess fat if desired.
2. Defrost frozen veggies, (don't cook them) chop to desired size.
3. In a large bowl mix cooked lamb, cooked rice, chopped vegetables, garlic and yogurt.
4. Slightly heat if desired to serve.
5. Refrigerate or freeze portions in Ziploc bags.

Makes three to six servings.

Doggie Doodle Biscuits

1 package active dry yeast
1 cup warm chicken broth
2 tablespoons molasses
1 3/4 cups all purpose flour — (1 3/4 to 2 cups)
1 1/2 cups whole wheat flour
1 1/2 cups cracked wheat
1/2 cup cornmeal
1/2 cup non fat dry milk powder
2 teaspoons garlic powder
2 teaspoons salt
1 tablespoon milk
1 egg — beaten

1. Dissolve yeast in 1/4 cup warm water, 110 to 115 degrees.
2. Stir in broth and molasses.
3. Add 1 cup only of the all purpose flour, all the whole wheat flour, cracked wheat, cornmeal, dry milk, garlic salt and mix well.
4. On floured board, knead in remaining flour.
5. Roll out 1/2 at a time to 3/8" thick. Cut in desired shapes.
6. Place on ungreased baking sheet, brush tops with beaten egg and milk mixture.
7. Repeat with remaining dough.
8. Bake at 300 degrees for 45 minutes.
9. Turn oven off and let dry overnight.

Makes 42 to 48 servings.

Fruity Yogurt Treats for Fido

2 kiwi fruit — mashed, or jar of baby food fruit
8 ounces strawberry yogurt — or other fruit flavor

1. Mix together,
2. Freeze in ice cube tray, serve.

Party Cake for Your Pooch!

Cake:
2/3 cup ripe mashed bananas
1/2 cup softened butter
3 large eggs
3/4 cup water
2 cups unbleached flour
2 teaspoons baking powder
1 teaspoon baking soda
2 teaspoons cinnamon
1/2 cup chopped pecans
1/2 cup raisins

Cake Instructions:
1. In a mixing bowl, beat together mashed banana and butter until creamy.
2. Add eggs and water. Beat well.
3. Stir in dry ingredients. Beat until smooth.
4. Add nuts and raisins.
5. Spoon batter evenly into oiled and floured bundt pan.
6. Bake at 350 degrees for about 35 minutes.
7. Cool on wire rack 5 minutes, remove from pan, replace on a rack and cool.

Frosting:
2 cups mashed banana
1 tablespoon butter
6 tablespoons carob flour
2 teaspoons vanilla
3 tablespoons unbleached flour
1 teaspoon cinnamon

Frosting Instructions:
1. Blend thoroughly and spread on cool cake.
2. Sprinkle with chopped pecans.
3. The frosting contains carob, which is a safe (almost tastes like) chocolate substitute.

Basic Dog Biscuits #1

2 1/2 cups whole wheat flour
1/2 cup wheat germ
1/2 cup powdered milk
1/2 teaspoon salt
1/2 teaspoon garlic powder
8 tablespoons bacon grease — or margarine
1 egg — beaten
1 teaspoon brown sugar
2 tablespoons beef broth — or chicken
1/2 cup ice water
6 slices bacon — crumbled, optional
1/2 cup cheddar cheese, shredded — optional

1. In a big mixing bowl, mix all the ingredients thoroughly to form a dough.
2. Roll the dough out with a rolling pin and use a cookie cutter to make shapes for cookies,
3. Bake cookies at 350 degrees for 20 - 25 minutes.

Bone Bonanza

1/2 pound ground beef — uncooked
1/4 cup chicken broth
1/3 cup black beans, cooked — mashed
1/3 cup cottage cheese
1 teaspoon soy sauce

1. Combine ground meat and chicken broth in a bowl.
2. Add the black beans and cottage cheese. Add soy sauce. Mix all of the ingredients together thoroughly.
3. Mold the mixture into bone shapes and place on a cookie sheet.
4. Bake for 45 minutes in a 375 degree oven. Let cool.

Magical Rice N' Hamburger

2 cups rice
1/2 pound hamburger meat
1 teaspoon vegetable oil
1 clove garlic
1/2 cup carrots or broccoli or spinach
4 cups water

1. Put all ingredients into a large pot.
2. Boil until done.
3. Cool off and serve.

Doggie Chicken Treats

2 chicken thighs — or white meat
1 stalk celery — sliced thick
3 carrots — peeled and halved
2 small potatoes — peeled and cubed
2 cups rice — uncooked

1. Place chicken pieces in large pot. Cover with cold water (5 -6 cups).
2. Add carrots, celery, and potatoes to water. Add salt to taste if you want.
3. Cover and simmer on low heat about two hours until the chicken becomes tender.
4. Add the rice, cover and cook over low heat for about 30 minutes until the rice is tender and most of the liquid is absorbed.
5. Remove soup from heat.
6. Pull the chicken meat off the bone, discard bones.
7. Return shredded pieces to pot.
8. Stir well. Let cool.

Store in the refrigerator or freeze.

Healthy Hound Dog Snacks

1 cup white rice flour	1/4 cup soy flour
1/4 cup egg substitute	1 tablespoon molasses (unsulphured)
1/3 cup milk	1/3 cup powdered milk
2 tablespoons safflower oil	

Preheat oven to 350 degrees.

1. Mix dry ingredients together. Add molasses, egg, oil and milk.
2. Roll out flat onto oiled cookie sheet and cut into dally bite-sized pieces.
3. Bake for 20 minutes. Let cool and store in tightly sealed container.

Doggie Salmon Treats

1 can salmon, canned, pink	1/2 cup chopped parsley
3 eggs — shells included	1/2 cup sesame seeds — ground in coffee grinder
1/2 cup flax seeds — ground in coffee grinder	2 cups potato flour — (2 to 3 cups)

1. Put these ingredients into a food processor, mix really well.
2. Pour potato flour through the opening (2 - 3 cups) while the motor is running until the contents form a ball like pie dough.
3. Remove the dough from the machine and place on a potato floured counter or board.
4. Knead more flour in until it resembles firm cookie dough.
5. Roll out dough into about 1/4 inch thickness.
6. Use a knife or pizza cutter to roll our long strips and then cut crosswise to make small squares or use a cookie cutter.
7. Bake on cookie sheets, sprayed with Pam or line the sheet with parchment paper.
8. Bake at 375 degrees for 20 minutes.
9. Rotate the cookie sheets and bake for an additional 10 minutes depending on how soft or hard you prefer to bake your treats.

Munchie Crunchy Meat Treats

1/2 cup powdered milk — non-fat
1 1/2 cups rice flour
1/2 cup water

egg — beaten
1/2 teaspoon honey
5 teaspoons chicken broth or beef

1 jar babyfood, meat, beef, strained — meat, any flavor

1. Combine all ingredients well. Form a ball.
2. Roll dough out on a floured surface. Cut out desired shapes.
3. Bake in a 350 degree oven for 25-30 minutes. Let cool.
The treats should be hard and crunchy.

Super Stew for Dogs

1 tablespoon olive oil
2 cups cabbage — chopped
18 ounces canned sweet potatoes
14 1/2 ounces canned tomato wedges — undrained
1 1/2 cups tomato juice

2 pounds beef
3 cloves garlic minced, up to 4
3/4 cup apple juice
1/3 cup peanut butter
6 cups cooked brown rice

1 teaspoon ginger root — up to 2 teaspoons, grated
2 cups green beans, frozen — cut crosswise

1. Heat the oil in a large skillet over medium-high heat. Cook beef.
2. Add the cabbage and garlic; cook, stirring, until the cabbage is tender but still crisp (about 5 minutes).
3. Stir in the sweet potatoes, tomatoes, tomato juice, apple juice, and ginger.
4. Reduce the heat to medium-low; cover.
5. Simmer until hot and bubbling, about 6 minutes.
6. Stir in the green beans and simmer, uncovered, for 5 minutes.
7. Stir in the peanut butter until well-blended and hot, about 1 minute.
8. Spoon over rice.

Bow Wow Biscuits

3/4 cup hot water or meat juice	1/3 cup margarine
1/2 cup powdered milk	1/2 teaspoon salt
1 egg, beaten	3 cups whole wheat flour

1. Combine all ingredients in a bowl and mix well.
2. Roll into small logs (approximately 3 inches long) and bake at 325 degrees for about 12 minutes or until golden brown.

Doggie Meat Loaf

2 1/8 cups water
2 cups brown rice
2 large potatoes
2 large carrots
1 1/8 pounds pumpkin
1 large onion
2 cloves garlic
3/4 bunch silver beet
1 cup whole meal pasta — or Soya pasta
2 cups rolled oats
1 cup whole meal flour
1 1/8 pounds mince (or liver or fish)
3 eggs

1. Boil the rice in water for 10 - 15 minutes.
2. Chop veggies or put them through the food processor.
3. Add veggies and pasta to the rice and cook for 10 minutes.
4. Turn off the heat and cool.
5. Add mince, eggs, herbs, rolled oats and flour and mix together. (Add more oats or flour if mixture is sticky (should be like a fruit cake mix)).
6. Spoon into oiled and floured loaf tins and bake at 350 for one hour.
7. Remove from tins. Turn oven off and return loaves to oven for 5 -10 minutes to firm bottom crust.
8. Remove from oven and cool.
9. Use immediately or wrap in foil and freeze. Makes 3 - 4 loaves.

Poochie Biscuits

2 1/2 cups Whole wheat flour
  1/2 cup powdered milk
  1/2 teaspoon salt
  1/2 teaspoon garlic powder

1 teaspoon brown sugar
6 tablespoons butter (cold)
1 egg — beaten
1/2 cup ice water

1. Combine the flour, milk, salt, garlic powder and sugar.
2. Cut in cold butter until mixture resembles cornmeal.
3. Mix in egg; then add enough ice water to make a ball.
4. Pat dough to 1/2" thick on a lightly oiled cookie sheet.
5. Cut out shapes with a cookie cutter or biscuit cutter.
6. Bake on cookie sheet for 25 minutes at 350 degrees.
7. Remove from the oven and cool on a wire rack.
8. To vary the flavor and texture, at the time the egg is added, add any of the following:

1 cup purred cooked green vegetables or carrots;
6 tablespoons whole wheat or rye kernels;
3 tablespoons liver powder. (The last two items are available in health food stores.)

Butter, margarine, shortening, or meat juices may be also used.

Lab Liver-Chip Cookie

2 cups whole wheat flour
1/3 cup butter — melted
1 egg — beaten
6 tablespoons water
1/4 cup liver — dried or jerky-style treats — chopped
Preheat oven to 350 degrees.

1. Combine flour, butter, egg, and water. Mix well.
2. Blend in liver bits.
3. Turn onto a greased baking pan. Bake 20 to 25 minutes. Cool and cut.

Biscuits With a Twist

1 envelope dry yeast
1 cup rye flour
1/4 cup warm water
1/2 cup nonfat dry milk
1 pinch sugar
4 teaspoons kelp powder
3 1/2 cups all-purpose flour
4 cups beef or chicken broth
2 cups whole wheat flour
2 cups cracked wheat or 1 cup cornmeal
Glaze: 1 large egg beaten with 2 tablespoons of milk.
Place 2 oven racks in the upper and lower thirds of the oven.
Preheat oven to 300 degrees.

1. Sprinkle dry yeast or crumble the compressed yeast over the water.
   Add a pinch of sugar and allow yeast to sit in a draft-free, warm
   location for 10 - 20 minutes. The mixture should be full of bubbles.
2. In a large bowl, combine all the dry ingredients and blend well.
3. Add the yeast mixture and 3 cups broth to the dry ingredients. Using
   your hands, in the bowl, mix to form the dough adding more broth if
   needed to make the dough smooth and supple.
4. Working with half a batch at a time, knead the dough briefly on a
   lightly floured counter. (Keep the remaining dough covered with a
   moist towel while shaping and cutting the first.)
5. Roll the dough into a 18"x13"x1/4" rectangle. Cut into desired shapes.
   Reroll scraps. Repeat procedure with remaining dough.
6. For an attractive shine, brush the glaze on the cookies before baking.
7. Bake for 45 - 60 minutes at 300 degrees or until brown and firm. For
   even baking, rotate cookie sheets from top to bottom racks after 25
   minutes.

Beef and Rice Moochies

1 jar babyfood, dinner, vegetables and beef, strained
2 1/2 cups flour, all-purpose
1 cup whole wheat flour
1 cup rice
1 package unflavored gelatin
1 whole egg
2 tablespoons vegetable oil
1 cup powdered milk
1 package yeast
1/4 cup warm water
1 beef bouillon cube (dissolved)

1. Dissolve yeast in warm water.
2. Mix dry ingredients in large bowl.
3. Add yeast mixture, egg, oil, babyfood and dissolved beef bouillon. Mix well.
4. Mixture will be very dry, knead with hands until it forms a ball. Roll out on floured surface to 1/4 inch thickness, cut in 1 or 2 inch circles.
5. Bake on un-greased cookie sheet 30 minutes at 300 degrees. Store in refrigerator.

Poochie Munchies

3	cups whole wheat flour	1	teaspoon garlic salt
1/2	cup soft bacon fat	1	cup shredded cheese
1	egg — beaten slightly	1	cup milk

Preheat oven to 400 degrees.

1. Place flour and garlic salt in a large bowl. Stir in bacon fat.
2. Add cheese and egg. Gradually add enough milk to form a dough.
3. Knead dough and roll out to about 1 inch thick.
4. Use dog bone cookie cutter to cut out dough.
5. Place on greased cookie sheet. Bake about 12 minutes, until they start to brown. Cool and serve.

Muttloaf

1/2 cup amaranth — *see Note
1 1/2 cups chicken broth
1 1/2 pounds ground chicken — or turkey
1/2 cup cottage cheese
2 whole egg
1/2 cup oats, rolled (raw)
1/4 cup carrot — finely chopped
1/4 cup spinach — finely chopped
1/4 cup zucchini — finely chopped
2 cloves garlic
1 tablespoon olive oil
Preheat oven to 350 degrees.

1. Add amaranth and chicken broth to sauce pan and bring to a boil, reduce heat and simmer for 20 minutes. Set aside and let cool.
2. In a large mixing bowl add meat, cottage cheese, veggies, and eggs. Mix thoroughly.
3. Add wheat germ, cooled amaranth and olive oil mix well.
4. Add mixture to loaf pan, bake at 350 degrees for 1 hour or until done.

Note: Amaranth can be found in a health food store, if not use barley. Barley will need 4 cups of broth and 50 minutes to cook.

Frozen Peanut Butter Yogurt Treats

32 ounces vanilla yogurt
1 cup peanut butter

1. Put the peanut butter in a microwave safe dish and microwave until melted.
2. Mix the yogurt and the melted peanut butter in a bowl.
3. Pour mixture into cupcake papers and freeze. Serve!

Liver Slivers

1/2 pound chicken livers — cooked	1 cup chicken stock
1/2 cup corn oil	1 tablespoon chopped parsley
1 cup powdered milk	1 cup rolled oats
1/2 cup brewer's yeast	1 cup soy flour
1 cup cornmeal	3 cups whole wheat flour

Preheat oven to 350 degrees.

1. In food processor or blender, process chicken livers, chicken stock, corn oil and parsley until smooth.
2. Transfer to large bowl.
3. Add powdered milk, rolled oats, brewer's yeast, soy flour and corn-meal. Mix well.
4. Gradually add whole wheat flour. You'll have to use your hands here, kneading in as much of the flour as it takes to create a very stiff dough.
5. Roll dough out to 1/4" thick and cut into stick shapes, about 1/2"by 4" (depending on the size of your dog). A pizza cutter works great!
6. Bake on ungreased cookie sheet for 20 to 25 minutes until lightly browned and crisp.
7. Turn off heat and let biscuits dry out in oven for several hours.

Store in the refrigerator.

Peanutty Pupsicles

1 ripe banana
1/2 cup peanut butter
1/4 cup wheat germ
1/4 cup chopped peanuts

1. Mash banana's and peanut butter, stir in wheat germ.
2. Chill 1 hour before serving.
3. Place in container, store in refrigerator or freezer.

Muttsa' Balls

1	cup natural dry dog food	2	eggs — beaten lightly
1	teaspoon cod liver oil	1/3	cup cold water
2	dashes garlic powder	1/2	cup cream of chicken soup or 2 bouillon cubes

1. Grind dry dog food smooth in a food processor or blender.
2. Lightly beat egg and add oil.
3. Mix all moist ingredients together except soup.
4. Add to dry ingredients.
5. Form into 1/2" balls.
6. In large pan, bring 1 quart water to a boil to which you have added 1/2 cup chicken soup or the 2 bouillon cubes.
7. Drop balls into boiling water. Boil for 3 minutes.
8. Remove from water, drain and cool. Refrigerate.

Potatoes Au Canine

3 cups boiled potatoes — sliced
2 tablespoons vegetables — grated
1/2 cup creamed cottage cheese
1 tablespoon nutritional Yeast
2 tablespoons grated carrots
1/4 cup whole milk
1/4 cup grated cheese

1. Layer in a casserole dish the first 5 ingredients.
2. Pour the milk on top of all; sprinkle with cheese.
3. Bake about 15 minutes at 350 degrees until cheese melts andslightly browns. Serve cool.

Notes: As a potato substitute, you can use 3 cups of cooked oatmeal or 3 cups cooked brown rice.

Peanut Butter & Oats Glazed Goodies

1 cup water	1 cup quick cooking oats
1/4 cup butter — half stick	1/2 cup cornmeal
1 tablespoon sugar	1 teaspoon salt
1/2 cup milk	1/3 cup peanut butter
3 cups whole wheat flour	

1. Boil water in a saucepan.
2. Add oats and butter. Let oats soak for ten minutes.
3. Stir in the cornmeal, sugar, salt, milk, peanut butter, and egg. Mix thoroughly.
4. Add the flour, one cup at a time (you may not need the entire amount) until a stiff dough forms.
5. Knead dough on floured surface until smooth, about 3 minutes.
6. Roll to 1/2" thickness. Cut into shapes. Place on a greased cookie sheet.

Glaze:
1 large egg beaten with 2 tablespoons of milk.
1. Mix well.
2. Brush glaze on dough with a pastry brush.
3. Bake in a preheated, 325 degree oven for 35-45 minutes or until golden brown. Cool completely before serving.

Special Meat & Grain Dinner for Doggies

2 cups cooked brown rice
2/3 cup lean beef
2 teaspoons lard — or veggie oil
1/4 cup vegetables

1. Mix the above. You can cook the meat if you want to, use your judgment.
2. Serve slightly warm.

Doggie Delights

1 ripe banana
1/2 cup peanut butter
1/4 cup wheat germ
1/4 cup unsalted peanuts — chopped

1. In a small bowl, mash banana and peanut butter together using a fork.
2. Mix in wheat germ.
3. Place in refrigerator for about an hour until, firm.
4. With your hands, roll rounded teaspoonfuls of mixture into balls.
5. Roll balls in peanuts, coating them evenly. Place on cookie sheet in freezer.
6. When completely frozen, pack into airtight containers and store in freezer.

Turkey Treats for Dogs

2 cups cooked turkey — cut up
2 cloves garlic
4 teaspoons grated cheese
1 tablespoon parsley — freshly chopped
2 eggs
2 cups whole wheat flour
2 tablespoons brewer's yeast
2 tablespoons vegetable oil

1. Combine turkey, garlic, cheese, parsley and mix well. Beat the eggs in a bowl and pour over turkey mixture.
2. Add the flour, yeast, and oil. Stir until thoroughly mixed and all ingredients are coated.
3. Drop into small lumps onto ungreased cookie sheet.
4. Cook in a 350 degree oven for about 20 minutes, until brown and firm.

Store in refrigerator.

Vegetarian Biscuits

2 1/2 cups flour
3/4 cup powdered Milk
1/2 cup vegetable oil
2 tablespoons brown sugar
3/4 cup vegetable Broth
1/2 cup carrots — optional
1 egg

1. Preheat oven to 300 degrees.
2. Mix all ingredients into a ball and roll out to about 1/4" thick.
3. Cut with bone-shaped cookie cutter, or strips, or a cutter shape of your own choice. Place on ungreased cookie sheet and bake 30 minutes.

Sunday Stew for Dogs

4 small parsnip
2 whole yellow squash — cubed
2 whole Sweet potatoes — peeled and cubed
2 whole Zucchini — cubed
5 whole tomatoes — canned
1 can garbanzo beans, canned
1/2 cup couscous
1/4 cup raisins
1 teaspoon ground coriander
1/2 teaspoon ground turmeric
1/2 teaspoon ground cinnamon
1/2 teaspoon ground ginger
1/4 teaspoon ground cumin
3 cups water

1. Combine all the ingredients in a large saucepan.
2. Bring to a boil, lower the heat, and simmer until the vegetables are tender, about 30 minutes. Serve over cook brown rice or barley.

Banana Bow Wow Bites

2 1/4 cups whole wheat flour
1/2 cup powdered milk — nonfat
1 egg
1/3 cup banana — ripe, mashed
1/4 cup vegetable oil
1 beef bouillon cube
1/2 cup water — hot
1 tablespoon brown sugar

1. Mix all ingredients until will blended.
2. Knead for 2 minutes on a floured surface.
3. Roll to 1/4 " thickness. Use a 2 1/2" bone shaped cookie cutter (or any one you prefer).
4. Bake for 30 minutes in a 300 degree oven on ungreased cookie pans.

Cheese & Veggie Poochie Chews

1/2 cup grated cheese — room temperature
3 tablespoons vegetable oil
3 teaspoons applesauce
1/2 cup vegetables — what ever you like
1 clove garlic — crushed
1 cup whole wheat flour
1 cup nonfat milk

1. Mix cheese, oil and applesauce together.
2. Add veggies, garlic, and flour. Combine thoroughly.
3. Add just enough milk to help form a ball. Cover and chill for one hour.
4. Roll onto a floured surface and cut into shapes.
5. Bake in a preheated 375 degree oven for 15 minutes or until golden brown. Let cool.

Cheese and Bacon Biscuits

3/4 cup flour
1/2 teaspoon baking soda
1/2 teaspoon salt
2/3 cup butter
2/3 cup brown sugar
1 egg
1 teaspoon vanilla extract
1 1/2 cups oatmeal
1 cup cheddar cheese — shredded
1/2 cup wheat germ
1/2 pound bacon — or bacon bits

1. Combine flour, soda and salt; mix well and set aside.
2. Cream butter and sugar, beat in egg and vanilla.
3. Add flour mix well, stir in oats, cheese, wheat germ and bacon. Drop by rounded tablespoon onto ungreased baking sheets.
4. Bake at 350 for 16 minutes. Cool and let the critters enjoy!

Cheesy Doggie Bites

1 cup wheat flour
1 cup cheddar cheese — grated
1 tablespoon garlic powder
1 tablespoon butter — softened
1/2 cup milk

1. Mix flour and cheese together. Add garlic powder and softened butter.
2. Slowly add milk until you form a stiff dough. You may not need all of the milk. Knead on floured board for 2 minutes. Roll out to 1 1/4inch thickness. Cut into shapes, place on ungreased cookie sheet.
3. Bake 350 degrees oven for 15 minutes. Let cool in oven with the door slightly open until cold and firm. Refrigerate to keep fresh.

Senior Doggie Cookies

3 jars babyfood, meat, beef, strained — *see note
1/4 cup cream of wheat — **see note
1/4 cup dry milk

1. Combine ingredients in bowl and mix well.
2. Roll into small balls and place on well-greased cookie sheet. Flatten slightly with a fork.
3. Bake in preheated 350 degree oven for 15 minutes or until brown.
4. Cool on wire racks and store in refrigerator. Also freezes well.
* **Note:** You can substitute carrot, chicken or beef babyfood.
** **Note:** You can substitute wheat germ for cream of wheat.

An Apple a Day Toto Treat

2 cups whole wheat flour	1/2	cup unbleached flour
1/2 cup cornmeal	1	apple - chopped or grated
1 egg — beaten	1/3	cup vegetable oil
1 tablespoon brown sugar, packed	3/8	cup water

Preheat oven to 350 degrees. Spray cookie sheet with vegetable oil spray. Lightly dust work surface with flour.

1. Blend flours and cornmeal in large mixing bowl.
2. Add apple, egg, oil, brown sugar and water; mix until well blended.
3. On floured surface, roll dough out to 7/8-inch thickness. Cut with cookie cutters of desired shape and size.
4. Place treats on prepared sheet. Bake in preheated oven 35 to 40 minutes.
5. Turn off oven. Leave door closed 1 hour to crisp treats. Remove treats from oven. Store baked treats in airtight container or plastic bag and place in refrigerator or freezer. Makes 2 to 2 1/2 dozen.

Apple Crunch Pupcakes

2 3/4	cups water	1/4	cup unsweetened applesauce
2	ablespoons honey	1	medium egg
1/8	teaspoon vanilla extract	4	cups whole wheat flour
1	cup apple, dried	1	tablespoon baking powder

Preheat oven to 350 degrees.

1. In a small bowl, mix together water, applesauce, honey, egg, and vanilla. In a large bowl, combine flour, apple chips, and baking powder.
2. Add liquid ingredients to dry ingredients and mix until very well blended.
3. Pour into greased muffin pans, Bake 1 1/4 hours, or until a toothpick inserted in the center comes out dry.

Store in a sealed container. Makes 12 to 14 pupcakes.

Bacon Balls

6 slices cooked bacon — crumbled
4 eggs — well beaten
1/8 cup bacon grease
1 cup water
1/2 cup powdered milk — non-fat
2 cups graham flour
2 cups wheat germ
1/2 cup cornmeal

1. Mix ingredients with a strong spoon;
2. Drop heaping tablespoonfuls in the shape of a ball onto a greased baking sheet.
3. Bake in a 350 degree oven for 15 minutes. Turn off oven and leave cookies on baking sheet in the oven overnight to dry out.

For both items, store in your refrigerator in an airtight container.

Barking Barley Brownies

1 1/4 pounds beef liver — or chicken liver
2 cups wheat germ
2 tablespoons whole wheat flour
1 cup cooked barley
2 whole eggs
3 tablespoons peanut butter
1 clove garlic
1 tablespoon olive oil
1 teaspoon salt — optional
Pre heat oven to 350 degrees.

1. Liquefy liver and garlic clove in a blender, when its smooth add eggs and peanut butter. Blend until smooth.
2. In a separate mixing bowl combine wheat germ, whole wheat flour, and cooked barley.
3. Add processed liver mixture, olive oil and salt. Mix well.
4. spread mixture in a greased 9x9 baking dish. Bake for 20 minutes or until done.
5. When cool cut into pieces that accommodate your doggy's size. Store in refrigerator or freezer.

Carrot Cookies

2 cups carrots — boiled and pureed
2 eggs
2 tablespoons garlic — minced
2 cups unbleached flour — *see Note
1 cup rolled oats
1/4 cup wheat germ
Note: or rice flour or rye flour.

1. Combine carrots, eggs and garlic. Mix until smooth.
2. Add dry ingredients. Roll out on heavily floured surface and cut into bars or desired shapes.
3. Bake at 300 degrees for 45 minutes or to desired crunchiness. The centers will continue to harden as they cool.

Bow Wow Burritos

1 tablespoon oil
12 ounces cooked beef — *see Note
1 clove garlic — minced
3 tablespoons chunky peanut butter
1 can sweet potatoes — (23-oz.) drained
1 can black beans — (15-oz.) rinsed
1 teaspoon chili powder
1 teaspoon cumin
1/2 teaspoon cinnamon
2 teaspoons beef bouillon — powder
6 flour tortillas — (10-inch)
2 tablespoons cilantro — chopped
6 tablespoons cheese — shredded
6 tablespoons vegetables — **see Notes below

1. Heat oil in large skillet over medium heat until hot. Add garlic; cook and stir 2 to 3 minutes or until tender.
2. Stir in peanut butter, sweet potatoes and beans; mash slightly.
3. Add cumin, cinnamon and chili powder, beef bouillon; mix well.
4. Reduce heat to low; add beef, cover and simmer 2 to 3 minutes or until thoroughly heated, stirring occasionally.
5. Meanwhile, heat tortillas according to package directions.
6. To serve, spoon and spread scant 1/2 cup mixture across center third of each tortilla with one piece of meat in center.
7. Top each with sour cream, cilantro, cheese spread to cover mixture.
8. Fold sides of each tortilla 1 inch over filling. Fold bottom 1/3 of tortilla over filling; roll again to enclose filling.

*Note: Beef or chicken cut into 1/2 inch strips, or "meatless" for the vegetarian doggies.
**Note: Shredded veggies for added nutrition; carrots, green beans, broccoli etc.

Marvelous Cookies

1 1/2 cups whole wheat flour
1 cup all-purpose flour
1 cup powdered milk - non-fat
1/3 cup bacon grease - *see Note
1 egg - lightly beaten
1 cup cold water

1. In a bowl, combine flour and milk powder. Drizzle with melted fat.
2. Add egg and water; mix well. Gather dough into a ball.
3. On floured surface, pat out dough. Roll out to 1/2 inch thickness. Cut into desired shapes.
4. Gather up scraps of dough and repeat rolling and cutting. Bake on ungreased baking sheets in 350 degree oven for 50 - 60 minutes or until crispy.

Note: Beef fat or Chicken fat can be used. Makes about 36 - 2 1/2 inch biscuits. Store in the refrigerator.

Mutt Munchies

1/2 cup nonfat dry milk
1 egg - well beaten
1 1/4 cups all-purpose flour
1 1/4 cups wheat flour
1/2 teaspoon garlic powder
1/2 teaspoon onion salt
1 1/2 teaspoons brown sugar
1/2 cup water
6 tablespoons gravy
2 jars babyfood, meat, beef, strained

1. Combine ingredients and shape into ball.
2. Roll out on floured board, Use extra flour if needed. Cut with knife or cookie cutter. Bake at 350 degrees for 25 to 30 min. Cool. Should be quite hard.

Cheesy Dog Cookies

2 cups all-purpose flour — un-sifted
1 1/4 cups cheddar cheese — shredded
2 cloves garlic — finely chopped
1/2 cup vegetable oil
4 tablespoons water — (4 to 5)

1. Combine everything except water.
2. Whisk in food processor until consistency of cornmeal. Then add water until mixture forms a ball.
3. Roll it into 1/2" thickness and cut into shapes.
4. Bake on ungreased cookie sheets about 10 min. (depending on size of shapes) at 400. Cool and store in refrigerator.

Canine Cheesy Carrot Muffins

1 cup all-purpose flour
1 cup whole wheat flour
1 tablespoon baking powder
1 cup cheddar cheese — Shredded
1 cup carrot — grated
2 large eggs
1 cup milk

Preheat oven to 350 degrees. Grease a muffin tin or line it with paper baking cups.

1. Combine the flours and baking powder and mix well.
2. Add the cheese and carrots and use your fingers to mix them into the flour until they are well-distributed.
3. In another bowl, beat the eggs. Whisk in the milk and vegetable oil. Pour over the flour mixture and stir gently until just combined.
4. Fill the muffin cups three-quarters full with the mixture. Bake for 20-25 minutes or until the muffins feel springy.
5. Be sure to let the muffins cool before letting your dog do any taste testing!

Chewy Cheesy Pizza for Doggies

Crust
2 cups cake flour
1 1/4 cups whole wheat flour
1/4 cup olive oil
1 egg
1 cup water
1 teaspoon baking soda

Crust Instructions:
1. Mix all ingredients together. Knead on a lightly floured surface.
2. Spray a regular sized, 12 " pizza pan with nonstick spray.
3. Next, spread the dough to the edges of the pan, forming a lip around the ends. Set aside.

Sauce & Toppings
1 tomato
1 cup tomato puree
1 clove garlic
1/4 cup parmesan cheese — grated
1/2 teaspoon oregano
1/2 teaspoon basil
2/3 cup cooked rice

Sauce & Toppings Instructions:
1. In a food processor, blend tomato, tomato puree and garlic.
2. Spoon the mixture over the pizza crust. Sprinkle the cheese and spices evenly over sauce.
3. Cut the pizza into slices with a pizza cutter or sharp knife.
4. Bake in a 325 degree oven for 25 minutes. Take out and sprinkle rice evenly over pizza.
5. Return to oven and bake 25 minutes more.

Yield: one 12 inch pizza.

Mini Cakes for Small Dogs

2 cups whole wheat flour
1/2 cup soybean flour
1 cup skim milk — or water
1 tablespoon honey
1 tablespoon canola oil — or sunflower
1 teaspoon sea salt

1. Mix dry ingredients.
2. Add liquid and honey.
3. Mix and let the dough rest in a warm place for 15 minutes.
4. Add oil and allow to sit another 1/2 hour.
5. Take walnut size portions of dough and flatten into small cakes.
6. Bake in oven at 400 degrees for 1/2 hour.

Fido's Birthday Cake

1 1/2 cups all-purpose flour
1 1/2 teaspoons baking powder
1/2 cup soft butter
1/2 cup corn oil
1 jar babyfood meat, beef, strained
4 eggs
2 strips beef jerky — (2 to 3)
Preheat oven to 325 degrees.

1. Grease and flour an 8x5x3 inch loaf pan.
2. Cream butter until smooth.
3. Add corn oil, babyfood, and eggs. Mix until smooth.
4. Mix dry ingredients into beef mixture until batter is smooth.
5. Crumble beef jerky and fold into batter.
6. Pour batter into loaf pan.
7. Bake 1 hour and 10 minutes. cool on wire rack 15 minutes.
8. Store uneaten cake in refrigerator.
Optional: Ice with plain yogurt or cottage cheese.

Doggie Quiche

4 whole eggs
1 tablespoon cream
2/3 cup milk, skim
3 ounces meat — *see Note
2 ounces shredded low fat cheddar cheese -or other type
1 whole pie crust (9 inch)
1/2 teaspoon garlic powder — optional
1 sprig parsley — chopped fine
Pre-heat oven to 375 degrees.

1. Wisk egg, cream, milk together, then pour into pie crust.
2. Add meat and cheese evenly.
3. Bake for 30-45 minutes or until done. Let cool.
4. Sprinkle fresh parsley.
* **Note:** fine chopped, any type of meat they like. Pre cooked, unless you use liver. Fresh shredded veggies can be used as well.

Wacky Wheat Treats

2 jars babyfood, meat, beef, strained
1/2 cup nonfat dry milk
2 ounces wheat germ
1/3 cup water
1/2 cup flour
1 teaspoon garlic powder

1. Mix together well. Roll out dough on floured surface.
2. Cut out witch hat patterns. Place on lightly greased cookie sheet.
   Bake at 325 degrees until golden brown, about 30-35 minutes.

Peanut Butter Swirls

Dough #1
4 cups whole wheat flour
1/2 cup cornmeal
1 1/3 cups water
1/3 cup peanut butter
1 egg

Dough #2

4 cups whole wheat flour
2/3 cup cornmeal
1/2 cup banana — mashed
1 egg
1 1/4 cups water
2 tablespoons vegetable oil
2 tablespoons molasses
2 tablespoons cinnamon

1. Combine all #1 ingredients and mix thoroughly.
2. Knead on a lightly floured surface. Set aside.
3. Combine all #2 ingredients and mix thoroughly.
4. Knead on a lightly floured surface.
5. Roll each dough separately to a 1/8 inch thickness, into rectangles.
6. Lightly brush a little water over the top of the light dough.
7. Place the dark dough on top, then roll up like a jelly roll.
8. Wrap the roll in plastic and chill in the freezer for one hour.
9. Cut the roll into 1/4 inch slices.
10. Place them on a cookie sheet sprayed with non-stick spray.
11. Bake at 350 degrees for one hour.

Scones for Spaniels

2 1/2 cups self-rising flour
1 cup beef liver - chopped *
1/2 cup water - or beef stock
1/2 cup milk
2 tablespoons butter
1/4 teaspoon salt

* Chopped Liver: Just boil the liver until it is gray and a rubbery consistency. Or if you have a microwave, cook it on high for about 8 minutes. Chop it up into small pieces and when cool put the pieces into a number of airtight bags and store in the fridge. Use liver pieces as treats when training.

Scones:
1. Sift flour and salt into a bowl, rub in butter.
2. Add chopped liver.
3. Use a knife to stir in milk and enough water to mix to a sticky dough.
4. Turn dough onto lightly floured surface, knead quickly and lightly until dough is smooth.
5. Press dough out evenly to about 2 cm and cut into rounds.
6. Place on a prepared tray and bake at 350 degrees for 15 minutes or until golden brown. Makes about 16-18.

Green Bean Mutt Grub

1 pound green beans — fresh or frozen, sliced
1 can cream of mushroom soup
1/2 cup milk
1/2 cup cheddar cheese — plus extra

1. Mix all ingredients together except beans.
2. Place beans in oven casserole, add sauce mixture and stir well.
3. Cover and bake in a 350 degree oven for 25 minutes. Uncover the casserole and sprinkle top with more cheddar cheese.
4. Bake 5 minutes more. Let cool before serving.

Walleye Dog Treats

3	pounds walleye pike fillets	2	ounces chicken livers — diced fine
2	cups fish stock	3	cups cooked brown rice
1/4	cup cooked wild rice	1/4	cup kale, frozen
1/2	cup green beans, frozen	1/4	cup collard greens, frozen
1/4	cup corn, frozen	1/4	cup potatoes, frozen
1	tablespoon cod liver oil		

Pre heat oven to 350 degrees.

1. In a baking dish add walleye fillets diced chicken livers, pour in fish stock and cod liver oil, add frozen veggies, cover and bake 20 to 30 minutes or until done.
2. In a large bowl add cooked rice, and the juices from the baking dish along with the cooked veggies, mix well.
3. Chunk the walleye into a size for your dog and mix well, if needed chop vegetables to a size for your dog.
4. Allow to cool and serve. Freeze leftovers or refrigerate.

Favorite Fido Cheesy Biscuits

1 1/2 cups whole wheat flour
1 1/4 cups grated cheddar cheese
1/4 pound margarine — corn oil
1 clove garlic — crushed
1 pinch salt
1/4 cup milk — as needed

1. Grate the cheese into a bowl and let stand until it reaches room temperature.
2. Cream the cheese with the softened margarine, garlic, salt and flour. Add just enough milk to form into a ball. Chill for 1/2 hour.
3. Roll onto floured board. Cut into shapes and bake at 375 degrees for 15 minutes or until slightly brown, and firm. Makes 2 to 3 dozen.

Divine Doggy Dinner

1/2 pound ground beef — or turkey, chicken, lamb
1/4 cup cooked rice
1 small potato
1/4 cup green beans — about 5-8 beans
1/4 teaspoon garlic powder

1. Brown the meat in a pan.
2. When completely cooked, drain the fat.
3. Add the cooked rice; mix well. Set aside.
4. Cut the potato and beans into small bite-sized pieces.
5. Place in a pot with water; bring to a boil.
6. Simmer until veggies are tender (about 15-20 minutes). Drain.
7. Add the vegetables to the meat mixture.
8. Add garlic powder; toss thoroughly under low heat. Let the dinner cool thoroughly before serving to prevent burning.
Yield: 2 dinners.

Crackers for Canines

2 1/2	cups whole wheat flour	1/2	cup dry milk — powder
1/2	teaspoon salt	1/2	teaspoon garlic powder
1	teaspoon brown sugar	6	tablespoons beef fat
1	egg — beaten	1/2	cup ice water

Preheat oven to 350 degrees and lightly oil a cookie sheet.

1. Combine flour, dry milk, salt, garlic powder and sugar.
2. Cut in meat drippings until mixture resembles corn meal.
3. Mix in egg.
4. Add enough water so mixture forms a ball.
5. Using your fingers, pat out dough onto cookie sheet to half inch thickness.
6. Cut with cookie cutter or knife and remove scraps. Scraps can be formed again and baked.
7. Bake 25-30 minutes. Remove from tray and cool on rack.

Peanut Butter & Honey Treats

3/4 cup flour

1 tablespoon honey

1/4 cup vegetable shortening

1/4 teaspoon salt

1/2 teaspoon vanilla

1 egg

1 teaspoon peanut butter

1 teaspoon baking soda

1/4 cup rolled oats

1. Heat honey and peanut butter until runny (about 20 seconds in the microwave.
2. Mix ingredients together and drop by 1/2 teaspoonful onto cookie sheet and bake at 350 degrees for 8 to 10 minutes. This normally makes 45 to 50 biscuits.

Oatmeal Poochie Biscuits

1 cup oatmeal — uncooked

1/3 cup margarine

1 tablespoon beef bouillon granules

5 1/2 cups hot water

1 tablespoon garlic powder — optional

3/4 cup powdered milk

3/4 cup cornmeal

3 cups whole wheat flour

1 whole egg — beaten

1. Pour hot water over oatmeal, margarine, and bouillon; let stand for 6 minutes.
2. Stir in milk, cornmeal, and egg. Add flour, 1/2 cup at a time; mix well after each addition.
3. Knead 3 - 4 min., adding more flour if necessary to make a very stiff dough. Roll or pat dough to 1/2" thickness.
4. Cut into dog bone shapes with cookie cutter. Bake at 325 degrees for 50 minutes on baking parchment.
5. Allow to cool and dry out until hard. Store in container.

Peanut Butter Cookies

2 cups whole wheat flour
1 cup wheat germ
1 cup peanut butter
1 egg
1/4 cup vegetable oil
1/2 cup water
1/2 teaspoon salt
Preheat oven to 350 degrees.

1. Combine flour wheat germ and salt in large bowl then mix in peanut butter, egg oil and water.
2. Roll dough out onto a lightly floured surface till about 1/2 inch thick, then cut out the biscuits using a cookie cutter - (or make squares).
3. Put the biscuits onto an ungreased baking sheet. Bake 15 minutes for smaller sized cookies and up to 35 minutes for larger shaped ones. Store in the fridge.

Beef Twists

3 1/2 cups flour, all-purpose
1 cup cornmeal
1 package unflavored gelatin
1/4 cup milk
1 egg
1/4 cup corn oil
1 jar babyfood, meat, beef, strained
1 beef bouillon cube
3/4 cup boiling water — or beef stock

1. Dissolve bouillon cube in water.
2. Sift dry ingredients in large bowl.
3. Add milk, egg, oil, beef and beef bouillon. Stir until well mixed.
4. Roll on a floured surface to 1/4 inch thickness. Cut in 1/4 inch by 3inch strips, twisting each stick 3 turns before placing on cookie sheet.
5. Bake 35-40 minutes at 400 degrees. Store in refrigerator.

Basic Dog Biscuits #2

3/4 cup hot water or meat juice
1/3 cup margarine
1/2 cup powdered milk
1/2 teaspoon salt
1 egg, beaten
3 cups whole wheat flour

1. Combine all ingredients in a bowl and mix well.
2. Roll into small logs (approximately 3 inches long) and bake at
   325 degrees for about 12 minutes or until golden brown.

Carob Covered Crunchies

2 1/4 cups whole wheat flour
1 egg
1/4 cup applesauce
1/4 cup vegetable oil
1 cube beef bouillon — or chicken
1/2 cup hot water
1 tablespoon honey
1 tablespoon molasses
1 cup carob

1. Mix all ingredients together until well blended.
2. Knead dough two minutes on a lightly floured surface. Roll to 1/4"
   thickness.
3. Bake on an ungreased cookie sheet for 30 minutes in a 300 degree
   oven. Cool.
4. Melt carob chips in microwave or saucepan.
5. Dip cool biscuits in carob or lay on a flat surface and brush carob over
   the biscuits with a pastry brush. Let cool before serving.

Homemade Liver Treats

1 cup whole wheat flour
1 cup cornmeal
1/2 cup wheat germ
1 teaspoon garlic powder
1 pound beef liver
Pre-heat oven to 350 degrees.

1. Liquefy liver in blender, add dry ingredients. Grease cookie sheet.
2. Drop teaspoonfuls of mixture onto cookie sheet and flatten with bottom of glass dipped in water and cornmeal. Bake for 15-20 minutes. You may store baked or unbaked dough in freezer.

Doggie Doodles

2 cups rye flour
1/2 cup vegetable oil
2/3 cup warm water
1/2 cup white flour
1/4 cup cornmeal

1. Combine all ingredients in a bowl and mix well.
2. Optional: I usually add about 1/4 teaspoon of either vanilla or mint flavor.
3. Roll out to 1/4" thick. Cut into shapes.
4. Bake on lightly greased cookie sheet for 30 minutes at 350 degrees.

Cat Treat Recipes

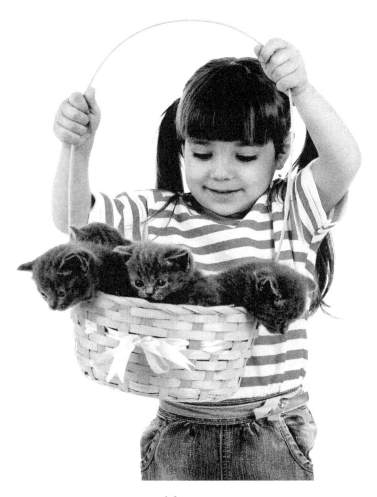

Beef And Veggie Broth

1/2 cup raw trimmed beef	3 tablespoons beef broth
2 tablespoons cooked oatmeal	1 tablespoon dried barley grass powder (find at a pet food store)

1 cooked minced veggie (Carrots are often a favorite)

1. Cook raw trimmed beef in just enough broth to cover, over medium to low heat.
2. When beef is cooked thru shred with fork and mix with the broth in which it was cooked.
3. Add the minced veggie and the barley grass powder. Stir well.
4. Last add the oatmeal to achieve the consistency that your cat likes. This is a good cat food recipe for indoor pets.

Better Than Grass Salad

1 small carrot peeled & grated	1/4 cup peeled and grated zucchini
1/2 cup chopped alfalfa sprouts	1 teaspoon finely chopped parsley
1/8 cup chicken stock	1/4 teaspoon dried or fresh catnip

1. Combine veggies in a medium bowl add chicken stock and toss.
2. Sprinkle with catnip and serve at room temperature.
3. Store leftovers in the refrigerator for up to 3 days.

Birthday Treat For Kitty

1 - 2 poached fish, (preferably salmon, with the skin and bones removed)
1 teaspoon plain yogurt
Few drops fresh lemon juice

1. Poach the fish.
2. Then mix the yogurt and lemon juice and serve over the cooked fish.
3. Allow to cool before serving

Kitty Kookies

1 cup whole wheat flour
1 teaspoon catnip
1/3 cup milk
1/3 cup powdered milk
2 tablespoons butter or vegetable oil
1/4 cup soy flour
1 egg
2 tablespoons wheat germ
1 tablespoon unsulfured molasses
Preheat oven to 350 degrees.

1. Mix dry ingredients together.
2. Add molasses, egg, oil and milk.
3. Roll out flat onto oiled cookie sheet and cut into small, cat bite-sized pieces.
4. Bake for 20 minutes and let cool. Store the cookies in a sealed container.

Kitty Krackers

6 ounces undrained tuna
1 cup cornmeal
1 cup flour
1/3 cup water
Preheat the oven to 350 degrees.

1. Measure all of the ingredients into a bowl and mix thoroughly with your hands.
2. Roll out to 1/4 inch thickness and cut into treat sized pieces.
3. Place on a greased cookie sheet. Bake for about 20 minutes or until golden.

Let cool and watch your cat gobble them up.

Jelly

3 cups chicken broth
4-1/2 tablespoon flour
1/4 cup carrots —diced into small cubes
3/4 cup minced meat (cooked) pieces of fish-optional, but it would be
  better to use this cooked.

1. After the chicken broth has been made, allow it too cool for around
   2 minutes.
2. Add all the flour and mix. Some flour might not dissolve but this will
   dissolve when you heat the mixture later on.
3. Heat broth and flour mixture on high heat until a thick creamy mixture
   is formed. Immediately add all other ingredients and pour all contents
   of this meal into the cat's container.
4. Allow it to set into jelly like substance with the carrots, minced meat
   and fish suspended in it. Serve.

Feline Hash

1 cup cooked ground beef   1/2 cup cooked brown rice
6 tablespoons alfalfa sprouts 3/4 cup cream-style cottage
                                      cheese

1. Mix together thoroughly and serve.

Cheese Please for Cats

1/2 cup grated cheese
2 tablespoons plain yogurt or sour cream
1/2 cup oatmeal
2 tablespoons margarine or low-fat spread

1. Mash all of the ingredients together, adding them in the order
   indicated above, and serve cold.
2. No cooking is required for this dish.
Some cats will not take to this dish as it is not meat based: others will
   love it.

Fabulous Feline Fish Balls

3 baby carrots, cooked until soft
16 ounces canned tuna in olive oil, drained
2 ounces cooked herring, skin removed
2 tablespoons whole grain bread crumbs or oatmeal
2-3 tablespoons grated cheese
2 teaspoons brewer's yeast
3 pinches of chopped catnip
1 egg, beaten
2 tablespoons tomato paste (not ketchup)
Preheat the oven to 350 degrees.

1. Mash the carrots with the fish, bread crumbs or oatmeal, cheese, brewer's yeast, catnip, egg and tomato paste to an even paste.
2. Mold into small balls and put on a greased baking tray.
3. Bake for 15-20 minutes, checking frequently.
4. The fish balls should be golden brown and feel firm. Cool thoroughly before serving.

Purrfect Chicken and Pasta Stew

2 packages ground chicken (or turkey)
2-3 small carrots, cooked
2-3 cups macaroni (cooked)
2 tablespoons vegetable oil
Garlic to taste

1. Boil the macaroni until tender.
2. Cook up the chicken in a frying pan.
3. Mix everything together in food processor.
4. Add the oil and the garlic. Mix well.

Chicken and Sardines for Cats

1 can sardines in olive oil
1/4 cup whole grain bread crumbs
1 egg, beaten
1/2 teaspoon brewer's yeast
2 cooked chicken drumsticks, bones removed

1. Drain the sardines, reserving the olive oil, and mash.
2. Mix in the bread crumbs, egg and yeast to an even, gooey consistency.
3. Coat the chicken drumsticks evenly in the mixture.
4. Heat the reserved olive oil in a frying pan then add the coated drumsticks and fry, turning frequently, until brown.
5. Remove from the heat, and cool before serving.

Purrrrfect Breakfast

3 eggs
2 tablespoons milk
3 tablespoons grated cheese
1 tablespoon margarine

1. Beat eggs and yolks together.
2. Stir in the grated cheese.
3. Melt the margarine in a frying pan until sizzling. Add the egg mixture, stirring continuously until cooked.

Finicky Feline Eaters Meal

1 cup chicken, boiled or microwaved
1/4 cup fresh broccoli, steamed
1/4 cup shredded carrots, steamed
Chicken broth as needed

1. Mix ingredients with enough chicken broth to hold together.
2. This same recipe can be used with fish (broil or microwave until it flakes). You can also vary the recipe by adding rice or other vegetables.

Chicken Cheeseburger

2	ounces finely ground beef	2	ounces finely ground chicken
1	tablespoon canned thick chicken soup	2	ounces whole grain bread crumbs or oatmeal
1	baby carrot, cooked until soft	1	egg
1/2	cup grated cheese		

1. Mash the meat and chicken with the soup then add the bread crumbs or oatmeal, mushy carrot and egg.
2. Make into two small burgers and broil (leaving much rarer than you would for yourself).
3. Sprinkle with grated cheese and broil again until the cheese is melted.
4. Allow to cool until warm to the touch, and serve.

Heavenly (Sardine and Rice)

2	cups flat cans of sardines in oil	2/3	cup cooked rice
1	tablespoon liver	1/4	cup parsley, chopped

1. Combine all ingredients. Stir with a wooden spoon to break up sardines into bite-sized pieces.
2. Store unused portion in refrigerator, tightly covered.

Kitty Kisses

1 can (or bag) cat food
1 Ziploc bag with the corner cut
3 pinches cat nip (optional)

1. Put cat food and optional cat nip in a blender or food processor and mix until it looks to be like frosting.
2. Put the mixture into the Ziploc bag and squeeze little droppings, or "kisses" onto a cookie sheet and bake in 300 degrees.
3. Time depends on how big the kisses are. Small are about 15 minutes. Cook thoroughly before serving!

Kitty Cat Chicken Soup

1 chicken liver
1 giblet
1 chicken heart
1 chicken neck
2 cups water
1 tablespoon finely chopped parsley

1. In a pot, combine chicken liver, giblet, chicken heart, chicken neck, water and finely chopped parsley.
2. Cover and simmer until the giblet is tender.
3. Removing bones grind the meat in the blender.

This can be served over your cat's normal dry food or on its own!

Chicken Crunchies

1-1/2 cups whole-wheat flour
1-1/2 cups rye flour
1-1/2 cups brown rice flour
1 cup wheat germ
1 teaspoon dried kelp or alfalfa
1 teaspoon garlic powder
4 tablespoons vegetable oil
1 1/2 cups chicken broth or beef broth
1 pound ground chicken
1 to 2 tablespoons brewer's yeast
Preheat the oven to 350 degrees.

1. In a large bowl, combine the first six dry ingredients.
2. Slowly add oil, broth and chicken, and mix well.
3. On a lightly floured surface, roll the dough to a thickness of 1/8 inch then place it on a greased cookie sheet.
4. Bake until golden brown. Cool then break into bite-size pieces. Place pieces in a bag with the brewer's yeast and shake to coat them. Store the leftovers in an airtight container in the refrigerator.
Makes 2 to 3 dozen pieces.

Crispy Trout Dinner

1   egg yolk
1   small trout fillet   3   tablespoons oatmeal
1   tablespoon vegetable oil

Preheat the oven to 350 degrees.

1. Beat the egg, dip the fish in it, and then coat it with oatmeal.
2. Put the oil in a small baking pan and lay the fillet in it, turning it over once or twice.
3. Bake for 15 minutes, turn over and bake for 15 minutes more.
4. Remove the fish to a dish, allow to cool.
5. Cut into bite-sized pieces.
Serving suggestion: if it looks a little dry, add a dash of cream.

Homemade Meal

1/4 pound liver (beef, chicken or   2   large hard-cooked eggs
       pork only)   1   tablespoon vegetable oil
  2   cups cooked white rice without   teaspoon potassium chlo-
       salt   1/8   ride (salt substitute)
  1   teaspoon calcium carbonate

1. Dice and braise the meat, retaining fat.
2. Combine all ingredients and mix well.
3. This mixture is somewhat dry and the palatability may be improved by adding some water.

Homemade Kitty Treats

1/2 cup dry cat food   1/4   cup warm water or milk
3   tablespoons catnip

1. Put the cat food and milk in the bowl and mix well. Pour out any extra water. Sprinkle the catnip over the mixture and mix well.
2. If you like you may bake in a 350 degree oven for 15 minutes.

Ham It Up Cat Treats

1 jar (2-1/2ounces) strained ham babyfood *Note
5/8 cup wheat germ
5/8 cup non-fat milk powder
1 egg, beaten
Preheat oven to 350 degrees.

1. Spray cookie sheet with vegetable oil spray.
2. Mix babyfood, wheat germ, milk powder, and egg in medium bowl.
3. Drop by 1/2 teaspoonfuls onto prepared baking sheet. Bake 12 to 15 minutes.
4. Remove from oven and let cool on wire rack. Store baked treats in airtight container or plastic bag and place in refrigerator or freezer. Makes - 2-1/2 to 3 dozen.
* **Note:** Beef or chicken babyfood may be substituted for ham baby food.

Catnip Cookies

1 cup whole-wheat flour
2 tablespoons wheat germ
1/4 cup soy flour
1/3 cup confectioners' milk
1 tablespoon kelp
1/2 teaspoon bonemeal
1 teaspoon crushed dried catnip leaves
1 tablespoon unsulfured molasses
1 egg
2 tablespoons oil, butter or fat
1/3 cup milk or water

1. Mix the dry ingredients together. Add the molasses, egg, oil, butter or fat and milk or water.
2. Roll out flat on an oiled cookie sheet and cut into narrow strips or ribbons.
3. Bake at 350 degrees for 20 minutes or until lightly toasted.
4. Break into pea-size pieces, suitable for cats. Good for treats, exercising gums and cleaning teeth.

Kipper Supreme

4 ounces cooked kipper
1 cup leftover cooked root vegetables
2 eggs
3 tablespoons milk
1/2 cup grated cheese
Preheat the oven to 325 degrees.

1. Mash together the fish and vegetables.
2. Put the mixture into an oiled baking pan. Beat the eggs, milk and cheese together, and pour on top of the fish mixture.
3. Bakefor about 20 minutes, until the outside is firm but the inside is reasonably soft. Remove from the oven and allow to cool.

Feline Cookies

1 cup whole wheat flour
1/4 cup soy flour
1 teaspoon catnip
1 egg
1/3 cup milk
2 tablespoons wheat germ
1/3 cup powdered milk
1 tablespoon unsulfured molasses
2 tablespoons butter or vegetable oil
Preheat oven to 350 degrees.

1. Mix dry ingredients together. Add molasses, egg, oil and milk.
2. Roll out flat onto oiled cookie sheet and cut into small, cat bite-sized pieces.
3. Bake for 20 minutes. Let cool and store in tightly sealed container.

Feline Treats

1-1/2 cups rolled oats   1/4 cup vegetable oil

  1/2 cup flour   1/2 cup tuna oil, chicken or beef bouillon

Preheat oven to 350 degrees.

1. Mix all ingredients into a dough.
2. Dust hands with flour and form small, 1/2-inch-thick, round "biscuits".
3. Set on greased cookie sheet.
4. Bake 30 minutes (or until biscuits are slightly browned).
5. Cool 30 minutes before serving.

Kitty Kat Biscuits

1 pound liver, organs, or other meat 2 cups old-fashioned oat-

2 cups bran   meal

                                    1/4 cup cooking oil

Preheat oven to 250 degrees.

1. Cover meat with cold water and bring to a boil. Immediately lower heat and simmer for 30 minutes. Remove meat from water and let cool; retain water.
2. When meat is completely cool, chop into 1-inch pieces and grind in food processor, chop in a blender, or process through a meat grinder until it is finely ground.
3. Mix ground meat, bran, oatmeal, and oil, adding the cooking water from the meat as necessary to make a thick dough. Avoid using any more liquid than needed to make a dough that is coarse and just wet enough to work with.
4. Shape the dough into small tiny flattened balls and arrange on an oiled baking sheet. Bake for 3 hours.
5. Then, turn off the heat and let the biscuits cool in the oven to ensure they are hard and crunchy. Let the biscuits air dry for 24 hours and store in an airtight container for up to 4 weeks.

Hint: Save organs from chickens, turkeys, etc. in a plastic bag in the freezer until you have enough to make this yummy treat.

Favorite Treats

1-1/2 cups cooked chicken or turkey
1 large egg
2 tablespoons chicken broth
1 cup cornmeal
1/2 cup whole wheat flour

1. In a blender or processor whirl chicken, egg and broth until smooth.
2. Scrape into bowl. Add cornmeal and 1/2 cup flour, stir until moistened.
3. Cover dough and refrigerate at least 2 hours. Then roll out 1/4 inch thick on lightly floured board.
4. Cut into 1/2 in squares or triangles. Scatter on 3 greased 12 x 15 baking sheets.
5. Bake at 350 degrees until golden for about 15 minutes.
6. Remove from oven, stir in pans and let cool. Refrigerate in an airtight container up to 2 weeks, freeze for longer storage.

Makes about 3 cups.

Kedgeree

1/3 cup white rice
1 tablespoon margarine or low-fat spread
3 ounce can tuna or smoked mackerel, skinned and boned
1/2 hard-boiled egg, shelled and finely chopped
1 yolk of the egg
1/2 tablespoon pouring cream

1. Cook and drain the rice. While the rice is cooking, gently fry the chopped tomato in the margarine until soft. Add the fish and the egg and continue cooking, stirring all the time with a wooden spoon.
2. Mix the rice, still over the heat, and stir everything seems steamy hot. Blend in the egg yolk, then the cream.
3. After a last few stirs, tip onto a plate and allow to cool.

Roll Ups

1	flour tortilla	1/8	cup chicken broth
1	cup ground chicken	1	teaspoon salt
1/8	cup cream (low fat)		

1. Mix up ground chicken with chicken broth inside a mixing bowl.
2. After mixed, pour chicken onto the middle of the tortilla.
3. Add 1 teaspoon of salt and 1/8 cup of cream on top of the chicken.
4. Roll up only two sides of the tortilla until they reach each other. Fold the other sides on top until they touch and serve to your cat!

Sardine Heaven

1	can sardines in oil	2/3	cup rice (cooked)
1/3	cup liver	2	teaspoons parsley and/or turmeric

1. Add all ingredients together.
2. You may wish to cook the ingredients, depending on whether your cats like fresh meat or cooked meat.
3. Store unused portion in fridge.

Mackerel Munchies

1/2 cup canned mackerel, drained
1 cup whole-grain bread crumbs
1 tablespoon vegetable oil
1 egg, beaten
1/2 teaspoon brewer's yeast, optional
Preheat oven to 350 degrees.

1. In a medium bowl, mash mackerel with a fork into tiny pieces.
2. Combine it with the remaining ingredients and mix well.
3. Drop mixture by 1/4 teaspoonsful onto a greased cookie sheet.
4. Bake for 8 minutes. Cool to room temperature and store in an airtight container in the refrigerator.

Smokie's Treats

1-1/2 cups rolled oats
1/4 cup vegetable oil
1/2 cup flour
1/2 cup tuna oil, chicken broth or beef bouillon
Preheat oven to 350 degrees.

1. Mix all ingredients into a dough.
2. Dust hands with flour and form small, 1/2-inch thick, round biscuits.
3. Set on greased cookie sheet. Bake 30 minutes or until biscuits are slightly browned.
4. Cool 30 minutes before serving.

Special Dinner

(good for cats with diabetes or kidney problems)
1 egg
1 tablespoon minced, cooked green beans
1 teaspoon shredded carrot
2 tablespoons baked chicken breast (no skin) minced
1/3 cup cooked brown rice (wild rice is good)
1 tablespoon olive oil (good for preventing hair balls and constipation - common to diabetics)

1. Mix all of the ingredients thoroughly with a wooden spoon or in a blender/food processor. It's important to get the rice mixed in well so that it can't be picked out.
2. (Diabetics need fiber and cats with kidney failure problems need to limit their protein intake so this serves two purposes.)
3. Cook in a small Pyrex skillet over low heat, stirring and "chopping" constantly, until the egg is at least soft-set but done.
4. Refrigerate in air-tight containers. Use within 36 hours (refrigerated). Stores well in the freezer in Ziploc baggies and can be thawed and warmed simultaneously in boiling water in the bag.

Liver Cookies

1/2 cup dry milk
1/2 cup wheat germ
1 teaspoon honey
1 (3 1/3 ounce) jar strained liver babyfood
Preheat oven to 350 degrees.

1. Combine dry milk and wheat germ; drizzle honey on top.
2. Add strained liver babyfood or homemade blended liver and stir until everything is well mixed.
3. Form the mixture into balls; place them on an oiled cookie sheet and flatten them with a fork.
4. Bake 8 - 10 minutes. Consistency should be fudgy.
5. Store in a jar in the fridge for up to 3 days or freeze.

Tuna Treats

1/2 cup whole wheat flour
1/2 cup nonfat, dry, powdered milk
1/2 can tuna, in oil (or 1/2 cup cooked chicken, chopped into small pieces
1 tablespoon vegetable oil or cod liver oil
1 egg, beaten
1/4 cup water
2 - 3 springs catnip (optional)
Preheat oven to 350 degrees. Grease cookie sheets with cooking spray.

1. In a large bowl, mash the tuna(or chicken)into smaller pieces.
2. Then add flour and milk. Mix well.
3. After all is mixed pour in water and oil. Mix well again.
4. Now, beat egg in a separate dish until egg gets a foamy texture.
5. Add to mix. Mix well. The dough will be sticky, so don't worry.
6. Using your fingers shape dough into small bite size balls, about the size of a marble. Put balls on greased cookie sheets.
7. Flatten. Bake for 10 minutes. Remove treats from oven wait five minutes and turn treats over so other side will cook. Bake 10 more minutes or until golden brown in color. Place treats on cookie rack to cool. Cool for 15 minutes before serving.

Mackerel Magic

2 slices unsmoked bacon, broiled
1 cup cooked brown rice
2 teaspoon soy sauce, Worcestershire or fish sauce
1 fresh mackerel, headed, tailed, cleaned and scaled

1. Chop the bacon up small and mix with the rice, adding the sauce in dashes as you go.
2. Broil the mackerel on both sides until crispy brown.
3. Allow to cool. Split along the stomach and gently open it out.
4. Bone, working from the head to tail.
5. Fill with the rice and bacon mixture, close over the sides of the mackerel and serve.

Meows

1	tablespoon oats	1/2	banana, mashed
2	tablespoons plain yogurt	1/2	cup orange juice
1/4	apple, chopped	2	ounces berries in season

1. Mix oats and bananas, blending well.
2. Add yogurt, orange juice and apple immediately to prevent browning.
3. Mash berries and add to mixture.
4. Serve in small portions (1 tablespoon per cat).
Note: too much fruit can cause diarrhea in a digestive system that is not used to it.

Tuitti Fruitti

1	teaspoon cantaloupe, minced	1	teaspoon watermelon, minced
1	teaspoon seedless grapes, minced		
		2	teaspoons cottage cheese

1. In a bowl, combine the fruit and cottage cheese.
Serve as a treat.

Mini-Cat Cakes

2 cups whole wheat flour
1/2 cup soybean flour
1 cup skimmed milk or water
1 tablespoon honey
1 tablespoon canola or sunflower oil
1 teaspoon sea salt

1. Mix dry ingredients.
2. Add liquid and honey.
3. Mix and let the dough rest in a warm place for 15 minutes.
4. Add oil and allow to sit another 1/2 hour.
5. Take walnut size portions of dough and flatten into small cakes. Bake in oven at 400 degrees for 1/2 hour.

Mouseburger Bites

3 ounces sausage meat or finely ground beef
2 tablespoons oatmeal
1 egg, to bind
1 teaspoon catnip, finely chopped

1. Knead the ingredients together thoroughly and form into a flat oval.
2. Broil under a medium heat for 5-7 minutes, turning frequently, until the outside is crisp.
3. Wait until cool, then slice into bite-sized chunks.

Honey Casserole

1 can tuna
1 teaspoon honey
1 serving cat's favorite food

1. Combine together and feed.

Smokie's Precious Treats

1 (12-ounce can) salmon with liquid   1   egg

1/2   cup flour   1/2   cup instant oatmeal, ground in a blender

1. Combine the salmon and egg in a blender; mix until smooth.
2. Add the oatmeal and blend well.
3. Spray cooking spray on a 9-by-13inch pan and spread the mixture in the pan. Bake at 350 degrees for 30-35 minutes.
4. Cool, then cut into bite-sized squares. Store in the freezer. Makes about 24 treats.

Potatoes Au Feline

3   cups boiled sliced potatoes   2   tablespoons grated vegetables

1/2   cup creamed cottage cheese   1   tablespoon nutritional yeast

2   tablespoons grated carrots   1/4   cup whole milk

1/4   cup grated cheese

1. Layer the first 5 ingredients into a casserole dish.
2. Pour the milk on top; sprinkle with cheese. Bake at 350 degrees for 15 minutes until cheese melts and slightly browns. Serve cool.
3. As a potato substitute, you can use 3 cups of cooked oatmeal or 3 cups cooked brown rice.

Tuna Balls

1 can drained tuna
1/2 cup cut turkey or chicken
2/3 cup dry cat food
1/2 cup sliced vegetables (optional)

1. Mix all ingredients in small bowl until well mixed.
2. Form into small balls or anything you're comfortable with.
3. Chill for about an hour.

Sardine Soup

2	cans sardines	1	pat of butter
1	cup water	5	stalks of watercress
1	teaspoon fish sauce (optional)		

1. Put the sardines and the pat of butter into a heavy-based frying-pan and place on a medium heat. As the pan warms and the butter melts, mash the sardines into it.
2. When the butter has completely melted, pour in the water and stir as it comes to a boil.
3. Thoroughly shred the watercress and toss into the pan. Remove the pan from the heat and allow to cool. Puree, and add a dash of fish sauce.

Sardine Surprise Treats

2	flat cans sardines in oil (do not drain)	2/3	cup cooked rice
1	tablespoon pureed liver	1/4	cup chopped parsley

1. Combine all ingredients and mix well.
2. Shape into balls of desired size or simply spoon into cat's dish and serve.
3. These treats may be stored in the refrigerator for up to three days, and may also be frozen.

Sautéed Liver

1	teaspoon corn oil	1/4	pound beef liver
1/2	cup water		

1. Heat 1 teaspoon corn oil in a pan.
2. Add 1/4 pound beef liver and fry on both sides until cooked but not dry inside.
3. Add 1/2 cup water to the pan and mix it up with all the brown bits. Grind the liver in a blender, using the pan juices.

Su-Purr Salmon Pate

1 (6 ounce) can boneless, skinless salmon
1/4 cup bread crumbs
1/2 cup finely chopped celery
1 egg, beaten
1 envelope unflavored gelatin
1/2 cup water
Preheat oven to 325 degrees.

1. Combine all ingredients and mix well.
2. Pack into a small fish-shaped mold (or other small mold) and bake for 45 minutes. Serve at room temperature.

Tuna Patties

1 can tuna
1/2 cup boiled rice
1/4 cup pureed liver
2-3 sprigs parsley chopped

1. Drain the tuna and mix everything together.
2. Make 6-7 balls and then pat them into patties.
3. Store in the fridge and serve to your cat. This is one cat treat recipe that your feline friend won't be finicky about.

Tuna Pops

1 can tuna packed in spring water

1. Drain liquid from tuna packed in spring water.
2. Freeze liquid in small ice cube trays (cocktail ice cube trays work nicely, as well as little square pill boxes available at most drug stores -- only fill these half full).
3. Give no more than 2 cubes at a time as a treat.
4. Reuse your can of drained tuna by placing in it an airtight container and covering with filtered water overnight for a second batch of tuna pop water.

Heavenly Sardine Surprise

2 flat cans sardines in oil (do not drain)
2/3 cup cooked rice
1 tablespoon pureed liver (or canned liver cat food)
1/4 cup chopped parsley

1. Combine all ingredients and mix well.
2. Shape into balls of desired size or simply spoon into cat's dish and serve.

These treats may be stored in the refrigerator for up to three days, and may also be frozen.

Kitty Kibbles

3	cups whole wheat flour	2	cups soy flour
1	cup wheat germ	1	cup cornmeal
1	cup nonfat dry milk	1/2	cup brewer's yeast
1	(15 ounce) can mackerel	5	tablespoons vegetable oil
1	tablespoon cod liver oil	2	cups water or as needed

Preheat oven to 350 degrees.

1. Mix all the dry ingredients in a large bowl.
2. In another bowl, mash the mackerel into small pieces. Mix in the oil and water.
3. Add the mackerel mixture to the dry ingredients and mix thoroughly. The dough is tough, so use your hands.
4. Roll dough out to about 1/4" thickness and cut into 1/4" bits, using a knife or pizza cutter. Mound the bits onto greased cookie sheets and bake for 25 minutes.
5. During baking, occasionally toss the bits with two wooden spoons, so they brown evenly.
6. Turn the heat off and allow the treats to cool thoroughly before removing and storing in an airtight container in the refrigerator. This recipe freezes very well for longer storage.

Homemade Yum Yums

1/2 cup dry cat food   1/4 cup warm water or milk
3 tablespoons catnip

1. Put the cat food and milk in the bowl and mix well. Pour out any extra water.
2. Sprinkle the catnip over the mixture and mix well. If you like you may bake in a 350 degree oven for 15 minutes. Cool before serving.

Catnip Tea

2 tablespoons catnip   1 cup water

1. Put the catnip in a bottle, pour in the water. Put the cap on the bottle, and shake until the catnip tea is green.

Diet for Divas

1 cup chicken, boiled or micro waved
1/4 cup fresh broccoli, steamed
1/4 cup shredded carrots, steamed
1/4 cup chicken broth

1. Mix ingredients with enough chicken broth to hold together.
2. This same recipe can be used with fish (broil or microwave until it flakes).
3. You can also vary the recipe by adding rice or other vegetables

Christmas Treats

1 cup minced leftover turkey   1/2 mashed cooked pumpkin
1 tablespoon oil   1 tablespoon kelp

1. Mix together and roll into balls. Feed as treats or give as x-mas presents for your kitty!

Yummy Cat Food

3 cups raw or lightly cooked ground meat (beef, chicken, turkey, or
    lamb)
1 cup raw or slightly cooked organ meat (kidney, liver, heart, lung)
1 raw turkey neck, ground or finely chopped (be sure not to cook)
1 cup well-cooked grain (oats, rice, barley or cornmeal)
1/2 cup well cooked vegetables (broccoli, zucchini, carrots, squash or
    green beans)
1 raw egg
1 teaspoon olive oil or flax seed oil

1. Mix all ingredients together, and then divide into individual portions.
2. The less you cook the ingredients, the more nutritional it will be for
   you cat. If you freeze the individual portions, they will keep for several weeks and you can defrost one a day.
3. When thawing, try not to use the microwave or another cooking
   method, since this will reduce nutrient levels. Instead, let food thaw
   overnight in the refrigerator. To warm it, place the food in a plastic
   bags with zipper closure, then immerse the bag into hot water for 10
   minutes.

Fish Delight

2 eggs
1-2 cups milk
2 tablespoons supplemental powder
1 tablespoon bone meal
1 tablespoon fresh raw veggies
1 tablespoon vegetable oil
1 can mackerel or tuna
4 slices brown bread

1. Blend together eggs, milk and then mix well with fish and bread.
2. Serve raw or bake for 20 minutes at 350 degrees.

Meat Majesty

1/4 can whitefish + tuna dinner wet cat food
1/4 can beef wet cat food
1/4 can chicken in gravy wet cat food
1/4 can salmon wet cat food
1/4 cup dry cat food

1. Mix together and feed. Put the rest in the fridge to keep fresh

Feline Frenzy

1/2 cup dry cat food
1 can wet cat food
2 teaspoon milk

1. Scoop the wet dinner in to Kitty's food dish and mush it up so it is in little pieces with Kitty's fork.
2. Pound dry cat food with potato masher in a Ziploc bag or run through your food processor. Sprinkle the pounded food onto the wet dinner.
3. Add milk and put into the microwave for 5 seconds and serve.

Cat Wrap

1 flour tortilla
1/8 cup chicken broth
1 cup ground chicken
1 teaspoon salt
1/8 cup cream (low fat)

1. Mix up ground chicken with chicken broth. After mixed pour the chicken on to the middle of the tortilla.
2. Add salt and cream on top of the chicken and then roll up the tortilla to serve.

Delight

1/3 slice bread   1/8 cup milk
1/8 cup chicken broth

1. Mix milk and chicken broth.
2. Tear the bread into tiny bits, then add to mixture.
3. Heat in the microwave for approximately 1 minute. When finished let cool, then serve to kitten

Grain Free Cat Food

1 pound ground turkey, chicken or beef
1/3 cup grated carrots
1/3 cup broccoli chopped in blender
1/4 cup liver puréed in blender

1. Mix all together. Put in ice cube trays and freeze. Take out and thaw as needed

Fancy Soup

1 hard boiled egg
1 raw egg
7 large pinches of garlic
1 capful olive oil
1 can tuna
1 cup water
rice
Don't use this recipe every day but it's great for those special occasions.

1. Mix in a bowl the hard boiled egg, garlic, olive oil, water, and as much rice as you want.
2. Squeeze the juice out of the tuna can and mix with other ingredients. Put in pan and bring to a boil.
3. Add raw egg and boil for 5 to 15 minutes and serve. (If your cat prefers a more moist dinner, don't drain the liquid out of the tuna before using.)

Cat Munchies

2 eggs
1 tablespoon milk
3 tablespoons cottage cheese
2 tablespoons finely chopped alfalfa sprouts
1. Mix all ingredients together.
2. Pour into a hot pan with a tablespoon of vegetable oil or butter.
3. When brown at bottom, turn over and brown the other side.
4. Chop into pieces and serve.

A + Dinner

1/2 carrot
1 serving cat food
1/8 cup milk
1 egg

1. First boil a half carrot. When it is soft, cut into small pieces.
2. In a separate bowl mix cat food, milk and egg.
3. Stir till mixed and then add carrots.

Beefy Goodness

1/2 cup raw trimmed beef
1 tablespoon beef broth
2 tablespoons cooked oatmeal
1 tablespoon dried barley grass powder
1 cooked minced veggies

1. Cook raw trimmed beef in just enough broth to cover, over medium to low heat.
2. When beef is cooked thru shred with fork and mix with the broth in which it was cooked.
3. Add the minced veggie (carrots are good with this one) and the barley grass powder. Stir well.
4. Last add the oatmeal to achieve the consistency that your cat likes.

A Lil' Ball of Love

1 can moist cat food
3 tablespoons milk
1/2 cup dry food

1. Mix the canned cat food and milk until sloppy.
2. Then add a dry food and mix.
3. For an added treat for your kitty you can add some tuna as well.

Chicken Stir Fry

1 diced raw chicken breast
2 tablespoons olive oil
2 tablespoons sliced almonds

1. Heat oil in wok or frying pan, and cook the meat quickly over a high flame, stirring all of the time.
2. When the chicken is almost cooked, stir in a few flaked almonds for added crunch.
3. Allow to cool and serve with a little plain boiled rice.

You Gotta Have Sole

1/2 pound fillet of sole
2 tablespoons onion, chopped
2 tablespoons parsley, chopped
to taste salt and pepper
as needed water
1 tablespoon butter
1 tablespoon flour
1/2 cup milk
1/4 cup cheddar cheese, grated
2 tablespoons liver
1/2 teaspoon iodized salt
2/3 cup cooked noodles, cut into kitty-bite-size pieces (or cooked rice)

1. Put sole in a small, greased baking disk. Sprinkle with onion, parsley, and a dash of salt and pepper.
2. Add enough water to just cover the bottom of the dish. Cook in a pre-heated 450 degree oven for 10 minutes.
3. Remove from oven, cool, and cut into kitty-bit-size pieces.
4. Melt butter in small saucepan.
5. Stir in flour and heat until bubbling.
6. Gradually stir in milk and cook, stirring constantly until mixture thickens.
7. Add cheese, liver, and salt; stir until cheese has melted.
8. Do not boil. Add chopped fish and noodles to cheese sauce and stir well.
9. Cool and serve. Yields 4 to 6 servings. Store unused portions inan airtight container and keep refrigerated.

Horse Treat Recipes

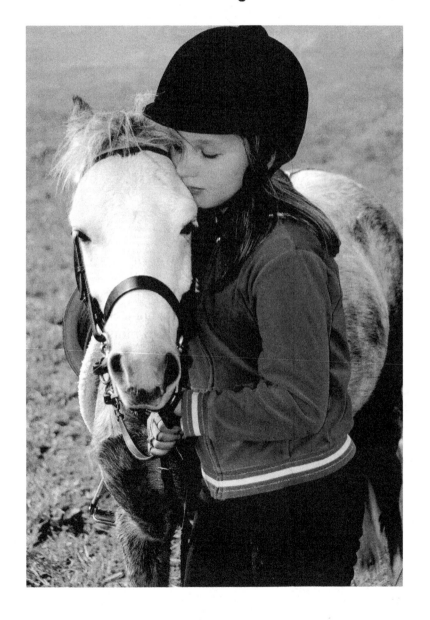

Cowboy Cookies #1

1 cup uncooked oatmeal
1 cup flour
1 cup shredded carrots
1 teaspoon salt
1 tablespoon sugar
2 tablespoons corn oil
1/4 cup water (one quarter cup)
1/4 cup molasses (one quarter cup)

1. Mix ingredients in a bowl in the order listed.
2. Make small balls and place on cookie sheet sprayed.
3. Bake at 350 degrees for 15 minutes or until golden brown.

Oatmeal Molasses Cookies

2 cups brown-sugar oatmeal (dry)
1/2 cup grated carrots
3 tablespoons molasses half cup brown sugar

1. Combine all these ingredients.
2. Add enough water to make into soft dough. Stir well.
3. Put into oven on 350 degrees for 10 - 15 minutes until golden brown
   and crisp.

Carrot Apple Delight

3 carrots chopped into small pieces
3 apples cut into small pieces
1 cup oatmeal

1. Drench cut up carrots and apples in molasses.
2. Roll molasses covered carrots and apples into oats, shake off excess.
3. Put in refrigerator for 30 minutes before serving.

Easy Cookies

1 cup carrots, grated
1 apple grated
2 tablespoons corn oil
1/4 cup molasses
1 teaspoon salt
1 cup rolled oats
1 cup flour
Preheat the oven to 350 degrees and lightly grease a cookie sheet.

1. In a large bowl, mix carrots, apple, corn oil and molasses together.
2. Fold in salt, oats and flour until well mixed.
3. Spread dough evenly in one piece on the cookie sheet.
4. Score dough with a knife to make it easier to break apart after baking
   (or use cookie cutters to make shapes!)
5. Let cool, break apart and serve!

Apple Muffins

1 cup flour
1 cup wheat germ
1/2 teaspoon cinnamon
1/2 cup white sugar
1/2 teaspoon salt
3 teaspoons baking powder
1 egg
2/3 cup milk
1/4 cup corn oil
1 cup apples, chopped
Preheat oven to 400 degrees.

1. Grease muffin tins and set aside.
2. In large bowl, mix dry ingredients together and set aside.
3. In separate bowl, mix remaining ingredients thoroughly.
4. Pour liquid ingredients into the dry ingredients. Mix until well
   moistened.
5. Scoop into muffin tins and bake 15-20 minutes.

Horse Cookies

1 cup uncooked oats
1 cup shredded Carrots
1 teaspoon sugar
1/4 cup molasses

1 cup flour
1 teaspoon salt
2 teaspoons vegetable oil

1. Mix ingredients in bowl as listed.
2. Make little balls and place on cookie sheet. Spray the cookie sheet with oil or Pam.
3. Bake at 350 degrees for 15 minutes or until golden brown.

Day Treats

1 packet Quaker Oatmeal (dry)
1 handful sweet feed
2 teaspoons applesauce
1 teaspoon honey or molasses
1/4 cup Cheerios
4 sugar cubes
1 tablespoon brown sugar
1/2 cup water

1. Mix the oatmeal with the water following packet instructions.
2. Add sweet feed and applesauce. Stir together.
3. Add the Cheerios, brown sugar, and honey or molasses.
4. Mix again and place sugar cubes on top.

Sticky Treats

1 apple or carrot
1/2 cup corn syrup
1 cup quick oats

1. Cut apple in half.
2. Remove core.
3. Roll in corn syrup then oats.
4. Do the same for a carrot and serve!

Birthday Cake

4 cups sweet feed or oats   1 cup molasses or honey
2 carrots cut into carrot sticks   1 apple cut into slices

1. Mix the honey and sweet feed or oats together in a big bowl.
2. When fully mixed, place the mixture on a plate and shape into the form of a birthday cake.
3. Use the carrots as candles and the apple slices as decorations.
4. Horses really enjoy this sticky but delicious treat.

Horse Muffins

1 1/2 cups bran
1 cup whole wheat flour
1 teaspoon baking soda
1 teaspoon baking powder
3/4 cup skimmed milk
1/2 cup molasses
2 tablespoons corn oil
1 egg, beaten

1. Stir together bran, flour, soda, and baking powder.
2. Mix together milk, molasses, oil, and egg.
3. Combine wet ingredients into dry ingredients.
4. Bake in greased or paper lined muffin tins at 400 degrees for 15 minutes.

Bonbons

1/8 cup molasses
8 crushed mints
4 carrots

1. Cut carrots into 1/4 inch pieces.
2. Drizzle molasses over carrots.
3. Sprinkle with mints.

Apple Horse Cookies

1 cup margarine
1 cup all-purpose flour
1 cup brown sugar
1 cup bran
1 cup diced carrots
1 cup diced apples
1 teaspoon baking soda
2 cups quick cooking rolled oats
2 eggs

1. Cream margarine and sugar until light and fluffy.
2. Beat in eggs.
3. Combine flour, bran and baking soda.
4. Blend into creamed mixture.
5. Stir in oats, carrots, and apples.
6. Drop by spoonfuls onto ungreased baking sheets and bake at 350 degrees for 10-12 minutes or until lightly browned.
7. Remove and cool. Makes about 4 dozen.

Mealtime Magic

1/2 apple
4 carrot chunks
1/2 cup molasses (or more if desired)
1/2 cup oatmeal (or more if desired)
1/2 cup warm water

1. Mix oatmeal and water together until it becomes warm mushy ball.
2. Sprinkle apple and carrots on top.
3. Pour molasses on top and serve.

Crispy Treats

1 1/4 cups rolled oats
3/4 cup dry oats
1/2 cup flax seed
1 cup molasses
1/4 cup flour
2 cups grain
2 cups water
Preheat oven to 350 degrees.

1. Soak 2 cups of grain with 2 cups water. Set aside.
2. Mix all dry ingredients together in medium to large bowl.
3. Drain excess water from soaked grain.
4. Mix molasses and soaked grain together in a small bowl, then add to large bowl with dry ingredients.
5. Form small, flattened patties and place on a cookie sheet.
6. Bake for 12 minutes (until well baked or a little bit burnt) so they are really crunchy after they cool!

Yummies

1cup flour
1/2 cup molasses
1/2 cup vegetable oil
1cup sugar
1/4 cup your horse's favorite treat (apple/oats/carrots/ peppermints crushed/grated)
Preheat oven for 350 degrees.

1. Mix sugar, flour, and crushed/grated goods.
2. Add liquids to sugar mixture. Stir until well blended.
3. The mix should be sticky, but not too runny. If it is too runny, add flour, if it is to thick, add a little more molasses and oil.
4. Form small disks and flatten to uniform size.
5. Bake for 10-15 minutes. Bake longer if necessary. Treats should be crunchy. Let cool in fridge before serving.

Apple n' Oaties

1 1/2 cups unsweetened applesauce
1 cup oat bran cereal or ground oatmeal
1/2 cup all purpose flour (approximately)
Preheat oven to 350 degrees and grease a 9 inch x 9inch square cake pan

1. Form a batter by combining all ingredients and stirring well.
2. Spread the batter evenly in the cake pan and bake for 20-30 minutes. When done, the batter will start to shrink away from the sides and it will be firm to the touch.
3. Slice into squares while still warm. Keep chewies in the refrigerator in an air-tight container or bag.

Molasses Treats

1 1/2 cups all purpose flour
1 cup bran
1 cup molasses
1 cup grated carrot or apple
Preheat oven to 375 degrees and oil two cookie sheets.

1. Put aside a small bowl of white sugar and a drinking glass with a flat bottom.
2. In a large bowl mix all the ingredients thoroughly. The mixture shouldn't be too wet, and should stick together.
3. Add more flour to make the mixture firmer if necessary.
4. Drop by teaspoonfuls, about 1 1/2 inches apart on a greased cookie sheet.
5. Grease the bottom of the glass, dip it in the sugar, and gently stamp the cookies to flatten them slightly.
6. Bake for about 10 minutes. This makes about 25 cookies, depending on the size. Store in an air-tight container or bag.

Banana Apple Treats

1 apple
2 bananas, very finely chopped
4 tablespoons honey
3 teaspoons powdered sugar

1. Cut the apples into slices, and spread the chopped bananas onto the apple slices.
2. Drizzle honey over the fruit, and sprinkle with powdered sugar.
3. Store in the refrigerator until hard. Serve.

Krispies with Carrot

2 carrots, shredded
1 apple, shredded
1/3 cup molasses
3/4 cup flower
1/2 cup brown sugar
1/2 cup water
3/4 cup bran
3/4 cup oatmeal
Preheat over to 400 degrees and generously grease a muffin tin.

1. Mix carrots and apples into a bowl with molasses, bran, brown sugar, water, flour and oatmeal.
2. Mixture should have a thick and doughy consistency. Add more bran if needed.
3. Scoop dough into a muffin tin, sprinkle each muffin with brown sugar and bake in oven for 30-50 minutes until well cooked.

Peppermint Treats

2 cups flour
1 cup oats
1/4 cup molasses
10 crushed peppermints
2 apples

1.Mix flour and oats together.
2. Add molasses if the mixture is not doughy.
3. Add water slowly until it is doughy.
4. Add peppermints and apples.
5. Cook for 8 – 10 minutes or until golden brown at 350 degrees.

Cowboy Cake

3 packages apple-cinnamon flavored instant oatmeal
1 cup flour
1/4 cup water
1/2 cup molasses
1 apple, cut into chunks
1 cup peanut butter
Preheat oven to 350 degrees.

1. Mix oatmeal, flour, and apple chunks together.
2. Then pour enough molasses to make a doughy texture.
3. Use an ice-cream scoop or your hands to make dough into balls. Flatten slightly to create a uniform size.
4. Place on a cookie sheet. Bake until golden brown 10 – 15 minutes – check regularly to avoid burning.
5. After cupcakes have cooled, spread peanut butter over the top for "icing."
If you find it difficult to spread, put the peanut butter in a microwavable bowl and microwave on high for 10 – 20 seconds. Keep a close eye on it!

Banana-Glazed Apple

1 apple   1 banana
1 cup ice cubes

1. Peel and cut banana.
2. Put into the blender with the ice cubes.
3. Chop and blend it together until creamy.
4. Cut the top off an apple and carve out the middle.
5. Fill the apple with the banana mixture.
6. Put top back on.
7. Pour the rest on top and over the sides of the apple. Serve.

Trail Mix Balls

5 chopped carrots in one inch pieces
1/2 cup molasses (or as much as you want)
2 cups oats or quick oats
2 cups grain

1. Soak carrots in water for 15 minutes.
2. After they have soaked, drain and place them in a large bowl.
3. Add molasses. Stir until carrots are completely covered with molasses.
4. Mix in grain. Add more molasses until grain is covered.
5. When you have done all the steps, roll them in the oats and form a ball.
6. Wrap the balls in foil and freeze them.
7. Thaw before serving.

Trail Mix

1/4 cup powdered sugar   4 teaspoons salt
1 cup Cheerios   1/2 cup uncooked oatmeal
1 cup hard corn   3 teaspoons brown sugar

1. Put everything in a Ziploc bag, close the bag, and shake for 10 seconds. Serve.

Birthday Cake

4 cups sweet feed or oats
1 cup molasses or honey
3 carrots cut into sticks and shreds
1 apple

1. Mix the honey and sweet feed or oats together in a big bowl.
2. When mixed fully together, place the mixture on a plate and shape into the form of a birthday cake or a carrot. Use your imagination.
3. Use the carrots as candles and garnish the rest of the cake with apple and carrot shavings.

Cowboy Cookies #2

1 cup dry oatmeal
1 cup flour
1 cup shredded carrots or apples
1 teaspoon salt
1 teaspoon sugar
2 teaspoons vegetable oil
1/4 cup molasses

1. Mix ingredients in bowl as listed.
2. Make little balls and place on greased cookie sheet.
3. Bake at 350 degrees for 15 minutes or until golden brown.

Apples Sweeties

1 apple, cored and chopped
1/4 cup honey
1 teaspoon cinnamon

1. Mix honey and cinnamon together in a small bowl.
2. Core and chop apple into larch chunks.
3. With a knife, spread honey and cinnamon mixture on apple chunks.
4. Refrigerate for one hour before serving. Store in the refrigerator.

Palomino Pie

3 sliced apples
2 teaspoons honey
8 peppermints, crushed
1 cup oatmeal, plain
3 teaspoons peanut butter
1/2 cup applesauce
Preheat oven to 350 degrees.

1. Mix honey, 1/2 cup oats, peanut butter, and applesauce in a bowl.
2. Stir and put in microwave for 45 seconds.
3. Spread apple slices in a baking dish.
4. Add mixture on top of apples.
5. Sprinkle peppermint and 1/2 cup of oats on top.
6. Bake for 20 minutes or until peppermint melts. Once the peppermint is melted, it looks strange; but your horses will like it.
7. Let cool until warm and sprinkle a little sugar on the top.

Chilly Crunchy Mix

1 apple sliced into small pieces
1/2 cup hard corn
1/2 cup uncooked oatmeal
3 tablespoons powdered sugar
1/2 teaspoon salt
1/2 cup grain or favorite treats
1/2 cup Cheerios
3 tablespoons syrup, honey or molasses

1. Mix corn, oatmeal, apple slices, grain, cheerios, and salt together.
2. Drizzle on syrup and sprinkle with powdered sugar.
3. Chill in refrigerator over night before serving.

Morgan Mare Munchies

1 cup dry oats
1 cup shredded carrots and apples
1 cup flour
1 teaspoon salt
1 1/2 teaspoons sugar
1/2 cup molasses
1/4 cup water
Preheat oven to 350 degrees.

1. Mix dry ingredients first then add everything else.
2. Bake for 10-15 minutes, or until golden brown.
3. Refrigerate until ready to serve.

Apple Stuffing

1 apple (cored)
1/2 cup molasses or honey
1 cup dry oatmeal

1. Core the apple and remove all apple seeds.
2. Cover it in molasses or honey, and roll it in a bowl full of dry oatmeal.

Store in refrigerator until ready to serve.

Molasses Baked Apple

1 apple
1 tablespoon molasses
3 tablespoons brown sugar
Preheat oven to 350 degrees.

1. Core and cut the apple in half, pour 1/2 tablespoon molasses on each
   apple piece, and sprinkle with brown sugar.
2. Place on greased cookie sheet. Bake at 350 degrees for 5 minutes.

Trakehner Treats

1 large apple
1/4 cup molasses
2 tablespoons honey
1/4 cup sweet feed
1/4 cup dry oatmeal
1/4 cup oats
1 shredded carrot

1. Cut off the top of the apple and set aside top.
2. Core the apple.
3. Hollow out some of the inside.
4. Take the molasses and the rest of the ingredients and mix them together in a bowl.
5. Pour the mixed ingredients into the apple and put the top back on.
6. Store in refrigerator if not fed right away.

Peppermint Patties

1/3 cup oats
1/3 cup grain
1/3 cup molasses
1/3 cup flour
8 – 10 peppermints

1. Mix all the ingredients except for the peppermints to create a dough.
2. Divide the dough into 8 equal pieces and create patties out of each.
3. Place patties on a non-stick baking sheet.
4. Before baking, Place a peppermint in the middle of each ball of the dough.
5. Bake at 350 degrees for 21 minutes. This makes about 8 patties.

Cheerio Snacks

1 cup finely crushed Cheerios
1/3 cup oats
1/2 cup grape juice
Preheat oven to 375 degrees.

1. Pour the Cheerios and oats into a bowl, mix well.
2. Add just enough grape juice to moisten the mix and make a little sticky.
3. Roll into 1/2 inch balls and place on a cookie sheet.
4. Bake for about 15-20 minutes.

Tasty Cookies

1/4 cup molasses
3 or 4 apples, finely chopped
1 cup carrots, finely chopped
2 tablespoons corn oil
1 cup flour
1 cup rolled oats
1/2 cup bran or grain of your choice, optional
Preheat oven to 350 degrees and lightly grease a large cookie sheet.

1. Mix apples, carrots, oil, and molasses.
2. Mix in oats and flour.
3. Either spread the mix on a cookie sheet and break apart after they are baked, or roll the dough out and cut into cookie shapes.
4. Cook for about 20 minutes and cool before serving.

Healthy Delight

1 big apple
12 baby carrots
3 sticks celery
2 pieces lettuce
1. Chop everything small, and put it in a baggie.
2. Store in the refrigerator. Serve within 1 – 2 days for best freshness.

Saddle Seat Snacks

1 cup oatmeal
1 cup whole wheat flour
2 tablespoons molasses
1/2 cup water
1/4 cup diced carrot
Preheat oven to 350 degrees.

1. Add ingredients in order listed.
2. Place batter in round balls on a greased cookie sheet.
3. Bake for 8-10 minutes. Serve when cooled.

Cowboy Carrots

1 carrot
1 golden delicious apple (You may use any type of apple,
1/2 cup molasses

1. Core apple.
2. Cover the inside of the apple in molasses.
3. Shove the carrot inside the apple hole.
4. Pour molasses into a large plastic bag and put in the apple with the
   carrot in the middle, inside the bag. Close the bag and shake very
   well to thoroughly coat the outside of the apple.
5. Wet hands and remove the apple from the bag and serve!

Pony Pizza

1 plain rice cake
1/4 cup applesauce
1 carrot, sliced
1 apple, cored and sliced

1. Spread some applesauce on the rice cake.
2. Arrange sliced apples and carrots on top of the applesauce and serve.

Special Bran Mash

2 cups of three different kinds of feed
1/4 cup rice bran, optional
1 tablespoon honey
2 cups water
4 peppermints
1/2 cup sugar
2 carrots, chopped
1 apple, loosely cut

1. Mix feed, honey, and water in a bowl and put in the microwave for 2 minutes.
2. Add more water if needed.
3. Add sugar, carrots, apples and mix well.
4. Add peppermints.
5. This mash can be refrigerated and reheated before serving.
6. Be sure that the mash isn't too hot before serving to your horse.

Nacho Treats

1 cup oats
1 cup water
1/3 cup molasses
1 tablespoon honey
1 carrot, shredded
10 crushed peppermints
Preheat oven to 350 degrees.

1. Stir oats, water, molasses, honey, and shredded carrots.
2. Let sit for 10 - 15 minutes.
3. Put all ingredients except peppermints on a greased pan, and bake for about 20 minutes.
4. Take out of oven and immediately sprinkle with crushed peppermint. Letcool before serving.

Cornmeal Cookies

2 cups quick oats
2 cups bran
2 cups cornmeal
12 ounces molasses
1 cup dark corn syrup
1/2 cup warm water
1/2 cup flour

1. Mix all ingredients together in either a large bowl or in a gallon sized Ziploc bag.
2. Let stand for 1 hour.
3. Shape into cookies using about 1 teaspoon of dough. If you mixed in a gallon sized Ziploc bag, you can snip the corner off the bag and pipe them onto your cooking surface, using a butter knife to cut them.
4. Place on a baking stone, and bake at 350 degrees for 20 minutes or until the edges are browning.

Apple Explosion

1 cup oatmeal
1 cup whole wheat flour
1/2 tablespoon brown sugar
2 teaspoons molasses
1/2 cup water
1/4 diced apple
Preheat oven to 350 degrees.

1. Mix all ingredients in order listed excluding the apple.
2. Grab some batter and stick a piece of the apple into the batter so it cannot be seen from the outside.
3. Do this to every cookie. Place them on a greased cookie sheet.
4. Bake for 8-10 minutes.

Oat Cookies

1/2 cup flour
1/4 teaspoon baking powder
1/4 teaspoon baking soda
1/4 cup oil
1/4 cup brown sugar
1/4 cup granulated sugar
1 tablespoon milk
1/4 teaspoon vanilla
1/4 cup uncooked regular oatmeal
1 1/2 cups grated carrots
Preheat oven to 350 degrees.

1. Combine all ingredients in a large bowl/gallon sized Ziploc bag.
2. Either roll dough into 1-inch balls and place on an un-greased cookie sheet or snip off the corner of the Ziploc bag and pipe them out using a butter knife to separate each one.
3. Bake for 15 minutes and cool for one hour.

Rockin' Cookies

1 cup oats   1/2 cup water
1/3 cup molasses   1 tablespoon honey
Preheat oven to 350 degrees.

1. Stir all the ingredients and let sit for about 10 minutes.
2. Scoop the mixture onto a lightly greased cookie sheet.
3. Bake for about 20 minutes. Let them cool.
4. They will look rubbery and burned, but they really are not.

Special Mash

1 packet instant oatmeal   1/4 cup molasses
5 baby carrots

1. Prepare the oatmeal per packet instructions.
2. Add all remaining ingredients.
3. Allow to cool before serving.

Yummy Biscuits

3 cups biscuit mix (instructions listed below)
1 or 2 carrots, coarsely grated
2/3 cup water
1/2 cup sugar
Hint: Make biscuit mix first
Preheat oven to 425 degrees.

1. Combine biscuit mix, carrots, and sugar in a large bowl.
2. Gradually add water to make a soft but not sticky dough.
3. Knead about 15 times on a floured surface.
4. Divide dough into 2 sections and roll each with a well floured rolling
   pin to 1/4 inch thickness.
5. Cut with a 2 inch round biscuit or cookie cutter.
6. Bake until lightly browned, about 8 minutes. Makes 40 biscuits.

Buckskin Biscuit Mix

10 cups flour
1 2/3 cup instant non fat dry milk
1/3 cup baking powder
2 1/2 teaspoons salt
1 2/3 cups shortening

1. Combine all ingredients in a large Tupperware bowl (8-10 quarts) that can be covered and refrigerated.
2. Add all ingredients and mix with a mixer very well.
3. Mixture should look like fine crumbs.
4. Store tightly covered in the refrigerator. It will last about 3 months. Makes about 15 cups of biscuit mix.

Bran Mash

1 1/2 cups uncooked oatmeal
1 cup Grape Nuts cereal
1/3 cup molasses
2 tablespoons brown sugar
2 tablespoons granulated sugar
2 tablespoons canola oil
2 tablespoons water
1 tablespoon vanilla extract
1 tablespoon peanut butter
1 package Oats and Honey bar, crushed
1 apple, chopped
1 carrot, chopped
1/8 cup flour
1 tablespoon cinnamon
Pinch of salt

1. Mix ingredients in a gallon sized Ziploc bag.
2. Let chill before serving, and only serve 1 cup, 2 – 3 times a week because it is very rich and could cause a belly ache if fed in too large a quantity!

Standardbred Surprise

2 tablespoons molasses   1 carrot, sliced
1 apple   3 tablespoons oats
2 teaspoons raisins   2 peppermints, crushed

1. Using a spoon, take the insides out of an apple. Be sure to dispose of the seeds.
2. Mix what you removed from the apple with all remaining ingredients except the peppermints.
3. Put the ingredients into the apple.
4. Sprinkle the peppermint pieces on top and serve.

Apple Cinnamon Muffins

1-1/2 cups apples, cut small
1-1/2 cups carrots, finely chopped or shredded
3/4 cup oatmeal, Quick Oats works great
1/4 cup apple juice
4 teaspoons molasses
1/2 cup flour
1 teaspoon brown sugar
1/8 cup cinnamon sugar

1. Cut apples and cut or shred carrots.
2. Use a few larger chunks of apple.
3. Add them in a mixing bowl with oatmeal.
4. Add apple juice, flour, brown sugar, and molasses.
5. Mix together. If runny add more oats. If it isn't sticky, add more molasses.
6. Put mix into a lightly greased muffin pan and bake at 350 degrees for about 8 to 10 minutes.
7. Take out one muffin at 8 minutes and see if it is cooked by inserting a tooth pick into the center of the cake. If the toothpick comes out clean, your cakes are done. If not, continue baking for 1-3 more minutes.
8. Let cool and dust with cinnamon sugar before serving!

Snacks

1 cup grated apple
1 cup grated carrots
1/2 cup oatmeal
1/2 teaspoon brown sugar
1/2 cup flour
2 teaspoons molasses
Preheat oven to 350 degrees.

1. Mix all ingredients well.
2. Spoon out small balls onto cookie sheet. Bake for 10 minutes, cool, and serve.

Peppermint Apples

1 large apple
1 shredded carrot
1/2 cup oats
1/4 cup honey
5 tablespoons sugar
1 tablespoon salt
3 crushed peppermints

1. Cut the apples in large chunks and set aside.
2. Mix the honey, peppermints, sugar, and salt in a bowl.
3. Mix the oats and carrots in a separate shallow bowl.
4. Coat the apple chunks in the honey mixture and roll in the oat mixture.
5. Place on a plate or Tupperware container and refrigerate until you feed to horses.
6. Keep refrigerated. Will store refrigerated for up to two days.

Kissey Cupcakes

1 cup cinnamon oatmeal
1 tablespoon wheat flour
1/2 tablespoon brown sugar
1/2 cup water
1/2 tablespoon honey
1 shredded apple
1/2 cup rainbow sprinkles

1. Core the apple, remove seeds before shredding. Set aside.
2. In a large bowl, mix the oatmeal, water, and honey.
3. Put the mixture in the microwave for about 2 minutes.
4. In a separate bowl, mix wheat flour, brown sugar, shredded apple, and extra ingredients.
5. Combine the contents of both bowls, and put this mixture in the microwave for about 2 more minutes.
6. Heat the oven to 375 degrees, and depending on oven they should finish cooking in 10 minutes.
7. Then add sprinkles, and let cook for 5 more minutes to get them crispy.

Favorite Snack Treats

1 cup baby carrots
2 apples, diced in big chunks
1 cup mini pretzels
2 1/2 cups molasses
1/2 cup honey
3/4 cup sugar
1/4 cup cinnamon
2 serving packages or 2 cups dry
oatmeal

1. Mix all ingredients together and leave on counter uncovered until it is room temperature. Serve.

Easy Trail Mix

1 apple   2 carrots
1 teaspoon sugar

1. Dice apples and cut carrots into medium sized pieces.
2. Add sugar and shake for 10 seconds.
3. You can freeze this mixture in the bag and slip it into your saddle bag as your head out on the trails. Makes a welcome treat for your horse!

Delight

1 large hollowed apple
1 1/2 - 2 tablespoons oatmeal, uncooked
1 1/2 tablespoons molasses
1 - 2 tablespoons grain
1 tablespoon brown sugar
1/2 grated baby carrot, optional

1. Mix together the oatmeal, brown sugar, grain, carrot and scoop into apple.
2. Drizzle molasses on the top. Serve.

Holiday Treats

1 cup flour   1 cup Grape Nuts cereal
1/4 cup light corn syrup (Karo)   1/4 cup water
2 tablespoons oil   1 teaspoon peppermint extract
3 drops food coloring (I use red)   Preheat oven to 350 degrees.

1. Mix all liquids and food coloring together in one large bowl.
2. Add dry ingredients and mix thoroughly.
3. Roll into balls or other shapes.
4. Bake for 15 to 20 minutes or until crispy.
5. Cool thoroughly before serving.

Healthy Cookies

5 strawberries
1 cup Golden Grahams (crushed)
2 1/2 cups Honey Nut Cheerios
2 1/2 cups flour
1 cup applesauce
1/2 cup crushed peppermints
4 baby carrots
2 cut apples
1/2 cup cinnamon
1/4 cup peanut butter
Preheat oven to 350 degrees.

1. Pour all ingredients into a big bowl, and mix well.
2. Shape into balls and place on a cookie sheet.
3. Cook for 15 to 19 minutes. Cool before serving.

Favorite Cowboy Cookies

1 cup apples, cut small
1 cup carrots, shredded
1/2 cup oatmeal
2 teaspoons molasses
1/2 cup flour
1/2 teaspoon brown sugar
Preheat oven to 325 degrees.

1. Mix everything really good, and put small balls of mix onto a lightly greased cookie sheet.
2. Bake cookies about 10 minutes.
3. Make sure the cookies are cooled before you serve them to your horse or pony.

Sticky Surprise

1/2 cup applesauce
1/4 cup molasses
1 small cut apple
4 chopped baby carrots, or 1 large cut
carrot if you don't have baby carrots
2 cups flour
2 cups Cheerios
2 strawberries
2 cups oatmeal
1 cup Rice Krispies cereal

1. Put all ingredients in a large bowl, and stir it together.
2. Form into small balls and place on greased cookie sheet.
3. Bake at 350 degrees for 15 minutes.
4. Let it cool for about 30 minutes before serving.

Surprise

1/2 apple (cut up in very small chunks)
1 cup malt o meal
3 tablespoons sugar
3 teaspoons cinnamon
2 tablespoons brown sugar
1/3 cup water
1/2 teaspoon salt
1/4 cup molasses
Preheat oven to 350 degrees.

1. Mix together all ingredients in order they are listed.
2. Grease cookie sheet, and make about 3/4 inch balls out of your mixture.
3. Place the balls on the sheet. Cook for 20 minutes occasionally checking on them.
4. Once finished, let cool with the oven shut off and the door slightly ajar for two hours.

Favorite Snack Treats

1 cup uncooked oatmeal
1 cup flour
1 cup shredded carrots or apples
1 teaspoon salt
1 tablespoon sugar
2 tablespoons corn or vegetable oil
1/4 cup water
1/4 cup molasses

1. Mix the ingredients into a large bowl in the order they are listed.
2. Make small balls and place on a greased cookie sheet.
3. Bake at 350 degrees for 15 minutes. Leave them in the oven after turning the oven off, until they are cool, and they will harden.

Icicle Treat

1 extra large carrot
1/2 apple cut in chunks (optional)
2 tablespoons peanut butter
3 tablespoons honey
2 teaspoons powdered sugar
1 tablespoon brown sugar

1. Hollow the carrot so that it looks like a small canoe.
2. Spread honey all over the outside of the carrot, and roll it in powdered sugar.
3. Spread the peanut butter inside the hollowed part.
4. Sprinkle brown sugar on top of the peanut butter.
5. To use apple chunks, scatter them on top of the brown sugar.
6. Drizzle honey on top of the brown sugar and serve.

Peanut Butter Oat Cookies

1/2 cup oats
1/2 cup water
1/4 cup peanut butter
1/4 cup whole wheat flour

1. Combine all ingredients except oats in a large bowl. Mix well.
2. The mixture should be the consistency of cookie dough.
3. If it is too thick, add more water.
4. Cut into shapes or roll into balls. Sprinkle oats on top, and bake at
   375 degrees for 15 minutes or until golden brown.

Pizza Treats

1 or more plain rice cakes
1/4 cup molasses
1 apple thinly sliced
1 carrot either thinly sliced or shredded
5 sugar cubes or peppermints

1. Coat the top side of the rice cake with the molasses and decorate like
   a pizza with any small treats your horse loves.
2. Coating only the top side of the rice cake makes it easier for you to
   serve!

Applesauce Treats

4 cups wheat flour
3 cups oatmeal
1 egg
4 tablespoons vegetable oil
1/2 cup molasses
4 tablespoons brown sugar
1 cup hot water
3/4 cup applesauce
Preheat oven to 300 degrees and grease a cookie sheet.

1. Mix oatmeal, flour, and brown sugar together.
2. Mix in the egg, vegetable oil, applesauce, and molasses.
3. Add hot water and mix well.
4. Roll out dough to 1/2 inch thickness on a floured surface.
5. Cut shapes using cookie cutters or make balls and flatten with a floured glass bottom to 1/2 inch thick.
6. Place on a cookie sheet and bake 1 hour. Turn oven off when they are done and leave the door shut until they are cool. This will make them crunchy.

Rice Krispie Snacks

1 box Rice Krispies cereal
1 apple or 1 carrot, diced
1 cup molasses
4 tablespoons sugar

1. Mix Rice Krispies, apple and molasses together. The mixture should resemble Rice Krispies Treats in consistency.
2. In a greased pan, flatten to about 1/2 inch thick.
3. Sprinkle with sugar.
4. Cut out with cookie cutters. Serve to your horse.

Yummies

1 or 2 sliced apples
1/2 cup baby carrots
1 or 2 cups corn
1 1/2 to 2 cups molasses
2 teaspoons apple juice
1 teaspoon sugar (optional)
1 tablespoon peanut butter (optional)

1. Slice apples and carrots into smallest pieces possible.
2. Put the first four ingredients in a mixing bowl and stir well.
3. Stir the last three items in well. Bake at 375 degrees for 10-15 minutes.
4. Turn the oven off and leave in the oven until cool.

Minty Molasses Sweets

1/2 cup molasses
12 peppermints
1/2 cup sugar
1/4 cup oats (optional)

1. Dip each mint into the molasses.
2. Place sugar and oats in a bowl and mix well.
3. Roll each mint in sugar and oats after dipping into the molasses.
4. Chill for one hour to firm up before serving.

Choice Treats

1 cup flavored or non flavored oats
1/2 or 1/3 cup water depending on consistency,
chewy or crunchy
2 to 3 baby carrots
1/2 cup raisins or small apple chunks
1 teaspoon butter
1/3 cup brown sugar

1. Mix all ingredients in a large bowl to form a dough.
2. Roll dough into balls or flatten and cut into shapes.
3. Place on buttered cookie sheet.
4. Bake at 350 degrees for 15 minutes.

Horse Muffins

3 cups oats
2 tablespoons honey or molasses
2 cups water
1 shredded apple
3 tablespoons flour
2 tablespoons brown sugar or white sugar
2 drops food coloring
4 crushed peppermints (optional)
Preheat oven to 375 degrees and grease muffin tins.

1. Core and remove all apple seeds before shredding apple. Set aside.
2. In a microwave safe bowl, combine oats, water, honey. Mix well.
3. Put in the microwave for 2 minutes.
4. Add shredded apple, brown sugar, crushed peppermints, food coloring, and flour.
5. Return to microwave for 2 more minutes.
6. The muffins will not rise. Bake for 15 minutes or until lightly brown.

No Bake Treat

1/2 cup peanut butter
2 large carrots
2 apples
1/2 cup sugar
1 cup oatmeal

1. Heat peanut butter in microwave until creamy. Start with 10 seconds at a time and keep an eye on it!
2. Grate carrots, chop apples (being careful to core the apple and remove the apple seeds).
3. Add all ingredients except sugar in large mixing bowl.
4. Mix together and sprinkle sugar on top of the treat.
5. Store in a pie plate or bowl in your refrigerator until you are ready to serve.

Cookie Magic

1/2 cup flour
1/4 cup oil
1/4 teaspoon baking soda
1/4 cup sugar
1/4 cup brown sugar
1 tablespoon milk
1/4 teaspoon vanilla
1/2 cup uncooked Quaker Oatmeal
17 baby carrots chopped very small
Preheat oven to 350 degrees.

1. Mix all the ingredients in big bowl.
2. Keep foil on un-greased cookie sheet.
3. Make the dough into about 1 inch balls. Makes about 17 balls.
4. Place on un-greased cookie sheet. Bake for 12-13 minutes.
5. Let them cool about 30 minutes. You can serve them as they are or place them in a gallon sized Ziploc bag and break them up into smaller pieces before serving. Store at room temperature.

Oatmeal Muffins

3 cups quick oats
1 tablespoon molasses
1 tablespoon honey
2 1/2 cups water
2 carrots, loosely cut
1 bag peppermints (optional)

1. In a microwave safe bowl combine oats, molasses, and honey. Mix well.
2. Add 2 cups water. Mix and put in microwave for 4 minutes. After 2 minutes, add carrots. Continue to cook.
3. Take out and heat your oven to 375 degrees.
4. In a greased muffin tin, add your mixture.
5. They won't rise, so fill them to the top.
6. Bake until the tops are lightly golden brown.
7. When done, remove and add a peppermint on top of each muffin. Serve when cool.

Tasty Pastry

1 cup oatmeal
1/2 cup molasses
1/4 cup sugar
1 teaspoon baking soda
2 shredded carrots
1 diced apple
1 cup water
1/4 cup smashed fruit loops
1 egg beaten

1. Mix all ingredients in a bowl. If dry, add more water. If watery, add more oatmeal.
2. Make into balls or shapes.
3. Bake at 350 degrees for 5 to 10 minutes or until golden brown.
4. Let cool for 10 minutes. Store in an airtight container.

Carrot Candies

3 large carrots
2 tablespoons brown sugar
3 tablespoons molasses
3 tablespoons raisins

1/2 small red apple
10 crackers, the dry, crunchy kind
1/2 cup Quaker Oats

1. Peel the carrots and cut them into chunks. Size really doesn't matter at this point.
2. Core the apple and cut into chunks.
3. Put the apple and carrot pieces into the blender and blend for a few seconds or until finely chopped.
4. Add the crackers and the Quaker oats and blend again until all the pieces are about the same size.
5. Add the molasses and brown sugar.
6. Blend again until fairly smooth.
7. Try to get it as smooth as possible.
8. If the mixture appears to be too dry, you may add a very small amount of fruit juice.
9. Grease a mini-muffin pan using vegetable oil (as horses are vegetarians).
10. Fill the tin with the mixture and if you like, top each "candy" with a raisin and freeze for 3 – 4 hours. Serve cold.

Note: Raisins could be substituted for peppermints if your horse prefers!

Copper Treats

15 mini carrots or 2 large carrots chopped
1 cup applesauce
1 packet Quaker instant oatmeal - regular

1. To make cookies, add a little bit of water to the oatmeal.
2. Mix all ingredients together and put on baking sheet.
3. Preheat oven to 350 degrees, bake for 10 minutes.
4. Store in a container at room temperature.

Delicious Cookies

1 cup oats
1/2 cup shredded carrot
1/2 cup finely diced apple
1 cup oatmeal
1/4 cup molasses
1/4 cup water
1 cup flour
1 teaspoon sugar
1/2 teaspoon salt
Preheat the oven to 350 degrees.

1. Stir the ingredients into a sticky mixture.
2. Roll the mix into balls with your hands.
3. About a heaping spoonful of the mixture makes each ball.
4. Grease a cookie sheet and arrange the balls on it.
5. Bake for 5 to 10 minutes or until golden brown. Let cool before feeding to your horse.
6. The treats can be stored at room temperature in an air tight jar.

Sugar Rush

1 apple
2 large carrots
1 tablespoon sugar
1 slice watermelon

1. Chop the apple into medium slices.
2. Cut carrots into small pieces. Store in a bag or Tupperware container.
3. Cut watermelon into small pieces. Put them in with carrots and apples. Add sugar.
4. Close bag or Tupperware, and shake until sugar isn't noticed. Serve.

Rice Krispie Bars

1 cup Rice Krispies
1/4 cup molasses
1/4 cup vegetable oil
1 shredded apple
2 teaspoons sugar
1/2 cup flour
1/4 cup water

1. Mix everything together in a bowl.
2. Make several rectangles with tin foil about the shape and size of a granola bar and lightly spray each with a non-stick cooking spray.
3. Pour mixture into the foil bar molds then set on a cookie sheet.
4. Heat oven to 350 degrees. Cook for 15 minutes or until they turn hard.
5. Take out of tin foil and place in the refrigerator overnight or for 30 minutes before serving.
6. Another option is to use non-stick mini-muffin pans if you find the foil sticks to the bars.

Molasses Treats

1 1/2 cups molasses
3 large carrots
2 apples
2 cups dry oatmeal

1. Slice carrots with cheese grader and mix well with molasses.
2. Slowly add the oatmeal and set aside.
3. Cut apples as small as you can, and add it to the oatmeal combination. Mix well.
4. Roll a little mixture at a time into a ball. Flatten like a cookie. Refrigerate for 2 hours.
5. Lightly sprinkle with sugar (optional).

Carrot Horse Cookies

2 cups feed (sweet or pellets)
2 cups shredded carrots or apples
1 cup molasses
Preheat oven to 350 degrees.

2 cups rolled oats
1 1/2 cups Raisin Bran cereal
1/4 cup brown sugar

1. Lightly grease cookie sheets.
2. Combine all ingredients and drop small spoonfuls on cookie sheet.
3. If mixture isn't clumping, add water and try again.
4. Cookies don't rise, so place as many on a sheet as possible.
5. Bake for 1 hour.
6. To get the crispiest results, after baking is done, turn off oven and let cookies sit inside the oven for another hour until oven is completely cooled.
7. These cookies are supposed to be hard and the recipe will make a lot of cookies for your horse. I suggest freezing some in an air tight container and refrigerating the rest in an air tight container. They will last a long time.

Healthy Equine Popsicle

1 cup carrot juice
1/2 cup apple juice
1/2 cup carrot bits and pieces and/or apple chunks
1 teaspoon sugar
2 long carrots (optional)

1. Mix carrot juice and apple juice together.
2. Add the sugar and mix until it has dissolved.
3. Add the carrots and apples.
4. Place in ice cube trays for bite sized pieces or put a long carrot in the center of a small bowl midway through the freezing process.
5. The carrot will act as a stick. Put in the freezer overnight. Serve cold.

Strawberry Treats

1 apple   1 large carrot
1 cup molasses   1 cup oats
12 strawberries

1. Shred the apple and carrot.
2. Chop the strawberries into small pieces.
3. Mix the shredded mixture with as much molasses as you think reasonable.
4. Mix in the strawberries.
5. Take a dab of the sticky mix, flatten it, and pat some oats on top. Put in refrigerator. Serve fresh and cold.

Early Morning Breakfast

2 carrots, well chopped
1 apple, well chopped and cored
1 handful sweet feed
1 handful pellets
4 sugar cubes
1/2 cup molasses

1. Mix the chopped carrots and apples with the sweet feed and pellets in a gallon sized Ziploc bag to avoid making a mess.
2. Soak the mixture with molasses. Seal the bag and manipulate the bag to coat everything thoroughly. If you need more molasses to coat, add more to the bag.
3. Freeze over night. I suggest laying the bag flat on a cookie sheet so the contents can spread out and freeze more evenly.
4. The next day, either open the Ziploc bag and deposit the contents into your horse's grain bucket or cut the bag open to remove the contents easily.
5. Place the sugar cubes on top and serve!

Bucket-Lickin' Treat

1 apple   1 large carrot
1/4 cup oatmeal

1. Cut up half of the apple and carrot. Put aside.
2. Shred carrot and apple. Leave a little bit of carrot and apple whole. Cut the last of the apple and carrot into fun little shapes if you wish.
3. Put apple/carrot treat into a gallon sized Ziploc bag, add 1/4 cup of oatmeal.
4. Shake well to coat and serve.

Sugar & Rice Krispies Coated Apples

2 apples, cored and sliced   1/2 cup sugar
1/2 cup molasses   1 cup Rice Krispies

1. Core and cut apples into about 5 slices each.
2. Put sugar and Rice Krispies in a big Ziploc bag.
3. Dip apple pieces in molasses and add to baggy.
4. Once all are added, zip shut and shake.
5. Empty bag to serve.

Veggie Goodies

1 apple
2 baby carrots
1/2 cup oats
1/4 cup sugar

1. Core and slice 1 apple into small chunks in a plastic Ziploc bag.
2. Cut 3 baby carrots and put them in the same bag.
3. Add 1/2 cup of oats and 1/4 cup sugar to the bag and shake.
4. Scoop and serve or empty the bag directly into your horse's grain bucket for a special treat!

Real Treats

1/2 cup molasses
1/4 cup water
3/4 cup whole wheat flour
1/2 cup oats
1 cup sweet feed

1. Pour molasses and water into a pot and turn on medium heat. Stir continuously until it starts to bubble but not boil.
2. After it bubbles, turn the heat on low.
3. Stir in the flour completely before adding and stirring in the oats.
4. Take off heat and quickly stir in the sweet feed.
5. Place on non stick cookie sheet or waxed paper.
6. It should be the consistency of cookie dough. Let cool and roll into balls to feed to your horse.

Apple Kisses

1 apple
1/2 cup white or brown sugar
1/2 cup oats
1/4 cup apple sauce
Preheat oven to 350 degrees.

1. Core the apple and cut into slices from top to bottom, creating large round slices. Set apples aside.
2. Combine oats, sugar, and apple sauce in a large bowl.
3. Avoid using too much apple sauce or else mixture will be too soggy.
4. Layout apple slices on a cookie sheet.
5. Take mixture and dribble over each slice so they are thoroughly covered.
6. Place cookie sheet in oven and bake for 5-10 minutes.
7. Take out, let cool, and serve!

Favorite Treat

1 apple
8 baby carrots
2 teaspoons sugar
3 tablespoons water
2 heaping tablespoons Quaker Oats (optional)
1 sandwich sized Ziploc bag

1. Core and chop the apples into medium or small sized cubes.
2. Chop the carrots into thirds or fourths.
3. Put the chopped ingredients into the bag.
4. Add the Quaker Oats, sugar, and water. Shake until all the ingredients are mixed thoroughly and serve.

Stuffed Carrots

1 apple
2 large carrots (not baby carrots)
1/4 cup sugar

1. Cut the ends off the carrots. Slice carrot into one inch long pieces.
2. Hollow out the carrots.
3. Core and dice the apples into very small pieces.
4. Dice the carrot centers and mix them together with the diced apple until it's a paste. You can use a food processor for this.
5. Roll the hollowed out carrot pieces in sugar.
6. Stuff the apple and carrot paste into the large carrot pieces and serve.
7. These can be stored in the freezer.

My Mare's Muffins

1-1/2 cup bran
1 cup flour
1 teaspoon baking soda
1 teaspoon baking powder
3/4 cup milk
1/2 cup molasses
2 tablespoons corn oil (it can be any vegetable oil)
1 egg, beaten

1. Stir together bran, flour, soda, and baking powder.
2. Mix in milk, molasses, oil, and the egg.
3. Bake in greased muffin tins at 400 degrees for 15 minutes.

Ice Cream Cones

1/4 cup applesauce   1 handful sweet feed
1 ice cream cone   1 teaspoon sugar

1. Combine applesauce and sweet feed in a bowl.
2. Place mixture into ice cream cone and sprinkle with sugar before
   serving.
Note: this is a great recipe if you are trying to hide pills that your horse
   would otherwise refuse to take!

Homemade Jerky

1 apple, cored   2 carrots
6 strawberries   1 cup oatmeal
1/2 cup molasses   1/3 cup sweet feed (optional)

1. Take the apple, carrots, and strawberries and dice them.
2. Put in a large bowl and add molasses. Mix well.
3. Then stir in oatmeal and sweet feed.
4. Put in the refrigerator for 30 minutes before serving.

Apple Snacks

1 large apple
1/4 cup bran
1/4 cup molasses
1 diced carrot (optional)

1. Core and hollow out a large apple as if it were a pumpkin.
2. Combine the diced carrot and apple meat you removed from the apple in a food processor until blended.
3. Add remaining ingredients and pulse a few times to combine.
4. Pour the mixture back into the apple and freeze overnight.
5. Warm it up in the microwave for about 30 seconds, slice it into several slices and serve!

Smart Snacks

1 packet instant oatmeal
1/2 cup oats
1/2 cup molasses
4 tablespoons peanut butter
4 tablespoons sugar

1. Mix oatmeal, oats, molasses and peanut butter together.
2. Form small balls and roll each ball in your sugar.
3. Refrigerate for at least one hour before serving.

Note: These are really handy to have around if you need to give your horse a pill or some other type of medicine they really don't like!

Carrot Horse Cookies

2 cups feed (sweet or pellets)   2 cups rolled oats
2 cups shredded carrots or apples   1 1/2 cups Raisin Bran cereal
1 cup molasses 1/4 cup brown sugar
Preheat oven to 350 degrees.

1. Lightly grease cookie sheets.
2. Combine all ingredients and drop small spoonfuls on cookie sheet.
3. If mixture isn't clumping, add water and try again.
4. Cookies don't rise, so place as many on a sheet as possible.
5. Bake for 1 hour.
6. To get the crispiest results, after baking is done, turn off oven and let cookies sit inside the oven for another hour until oven is completely cooled.
7. These cookies are supposed to be hard and the recipe will make a lot of cookies for your horse. I suggest freezing some in an air tight container and refrigerating the rest in an air tight container. They will last a long time.

Special Mash

1 packet instant oatmeal
1/4 cup molasses
5 baby carrots

1. Prepare the oatmeal per packet instructions.
2. Add all remaining ingredients.
3. Allow to cool before serving.

Sugar & Rice Krispies Coated Apples

apples, cored and sliced
1/2 cup sugar
1/2 cup molasses
1 cup Rice Krispies

1. Core and cut apples into about 5 slices each.
2. Put sugar and Rice Krispies in a big Ziploc bag.
3. Dip apple pieces in molasses and add to baggy.
4. Once all are added, zip shut and shake.
5. Empty bag to serve.

Copper Treats

15 mini carrots or 2 large carrots chopped 1 cup applesauce 1 packet Quaker instant oatmeal - regular

1. To make cookies, add a little bit of water to the oatmeal.
2. Mix all ingredients together and put on baking sheet.
3. Preheat oven to 350 degrees, bake for 10 minutes.
4. Store in a container at room temperature.

Thank you for Supporting Your Favorite Animal-Related Organizations!

Help for Non-Profit Organizations

If you are working with a non-proift organization, looking for fundraising ideas, visit our website at:

ttp://funding101.org

Our site is filled with helpful articles and loads of tips. While you are there, check out our digital program,

Making Profits for Your Non-Profit

The program includes more than:
* 100 fund raising and success tips
* 3 hours of audio files
* A 90+ page workbook
* AND,several FREE ADDED BONUSES

BONUS

When you get your **Making Profits for Your Non-Profit** program at http://funding101.org, we are including several FREE Bonuses:
* Our Audio interview with a grant writing expert
* Our Audio interview with a PR master explaining how to
* get thousands of dollars in free press
* Free Volunteer appreciation certificates you can print off and personalize as a thank you for all your volunteers

99% of the techniques taught in the program won't cost you a dime to implement but they are already costing you thousands in lost revenue until you do!
Purchase **Making Profits for Your Non-Profit** program today at http://funding101.org, and download the program immediately.

52312951R00076

Made in the USA
Middletown, DE
09 July 2019